Netter's Atlas of Human Physiology

Netter's Atlas of Human Physiology

John T. Hansen, Ph.D.

University of Rochester School of Medicine and Dentistry

Bruce M. Koeppen, M.D., Ph.D.

University of Connecticut School of Medicine

Illustrations by Frank H. Netter, M.D.

Contributing Illustrators

John A. Craig, M.D.

Carlos A. G. Machado, M.D.

James A. Perkins, M.S., M.F.A.

Icon Learning Systems · Teterboro, New Jersey

Published by Icon Learning Systems LLC, a subsidiary of MediMedia USA, Inc.
Copyright © 2002 MediMedia, Inc.

FIRST EDITION

ISBN 1-929007-01-9
Library of Congress Catalog No: 2001132797

Printed in the U.S.A.
First Printing, 2002

NOTICE

Executive Editor: Paul Kelly
Editorial Director: Greg Otis
Managing Editor: Jennifer Surich
Print Production Manager: Jim O'Keeffe
Art Production Manager: Michelle Jahn
Art Director: Joanie Krupinski
Cover Designer: Erika Gehringer

Binding and Printing by Webcrafters
Color Corrections by Page Imaging
Digital Separations by R.R. Donnelley and Page Imaging
Composition and Layout by Graphic World Inc.

We dedicate this book to our families,

and especially our spouses,

Paula Hansen *and* Dr. Christine Niekrash.

Their encouragement and support has been unconditional.

Preface

Netter's Atlas of Human Physiology is intended to provide the student of physiology a clear, concise, and user-friendly summary and review of the major principles of organ system physiology. The primary perspective is illustrative and represents a "view from 30,000 feet." We selected this approach predicated on the idea that once students see the "big picture," they are better prepared to layer on the necessary detail that ultimately completes their understanding. Accordingly, to attain the full value of this *Atlas,* it should be used as a supplement to, and not a substitute for, a comprehensive textbook of physiology.

Organized by systems, each chapter begins with the structure-function relationships of the whole organ or system and then moves the learner down the ladder of tissues and cells to the subcellular elements, highlighting at each level the physiology inherent to that level of organization. Graphs, tables, and schematics are used to quantitatively illustrate key concepts and summarize integrated relationships. As a supplement to a more comprehensive textbook, monograph, or course syllabus, this *Atlas* best serves as an initial introduction to new material and as a review after appropriate detail has been mastered. Consequently, this *Atlas* is an appropriate learning tool for students engaged in their first human or mammalian physiology course and as a review *Atlas* for students, physicians, and other health care professions who have completed such a course.

The obvious choice for the artwork used in this *Atlas* is the beautifully conceived and executed medical illustrations of the renowned physician-artist, Frank H. Netter, M.D. Dr. Netter's 45-year collaboration with the CIBA Pharmaceutical Company (now Novartis Pharmaceuticals) has produced a wealth of medical art familiar to physicians and other health care professionals worldwide. Dr. Netter's unique perspective and understanding of structure-function relationships renders his illustrations ideal for visualizing cellular and organ system processes in a manner that highlights the essential points and facilitates comprehension. His judicious eye for excluding detail that obscures while retaining that which is essential provides a view in natural harmony with our stated objective of presenting important principles in an overview format. Dr. Netter's plates, in the words of his friend and physician-artist colleague John A. Craig, M.D., "clarify" rather than "intimidate," while still maintaining "their technical accuracy and high artistic standards." Dr. Netter's images serve as the starting point for the plates in this *Atlas*. As necessary, these images were updated and supplemented by Jim Perkins, M.S., M.F.A., Dr. Craig, and Carlos Machado, M.D. The end result, we believe, is an illustration that provides a "clear picture of how the subject *is,*" rather than simply a drawing that shows only "how that subject *appears.*" Integrated structure and function come "alive" in these beautifully rendered color drawings and schematics, naturally enhancing understanding and learning. We hope that students will enjoy using this *Atlas* as much as we have enjoyed producing it.

John T. Hansen, Ph.D.
Bruce M. Koeppen, M.D., Ph.D.

Frank H. Netter, M.D.

Frank H. Netter was born in 1906 in New York City. He studied art at the Art Student's League and the National Academy of Design before entering medical school at New York University, where he received his M.D. degree in 1931. During his student years, Dr. Netter's notebook sketches attracted the attention of the medical faculty and other physicians, allowing him to augment his income by illustrating articles and textbooks. He continued illustrating as a sideline after establishing a surgical practice in 1933, but he ultimately opted to give up his practice in favor of a full-time commitment to art. After service in the United States Army during World War II, Dr. Netter began his long collaboration with the CIBA Pharmaceutical Company (now Novartis Pharmaceuticals). This 45-year partnership resulted in the production of the extraordinary collection of medical art so familiar to physicians and other medical professionals worldwide.

Icon Learning Systems acquired the Netter Collection in July 2000 and continues to update Dr. Netter's original paintings and to add newly commissioned paintings by artists trained in the style of Dr. Netter.

Dr. Netter's works are among the finest examples of the use of illustration in the teaching of medical concepts. The 13-book Netter Collection of Medical Illustrations, which includes the greater part of the more than 20,000 paintings created by Dr. Netter, became and remains one of the most famous medical works ever published. The Netter Atlas of Human Anatomy, first published in 1989, presents the anatomical paintings from the Netter Collection. Now translated into 11 languages, it is the anatomy atlas of choice among medical and health professions students the world over.

The Netter illustrations are appreciated not only for their aesthetic qualities, but more importantly, for their intellectual content. As Dr. Netter wrote in 1949, ". . . clarification of a subject is the aim and goal of illustration. No matter how beautifully painted, how delicately and subtly rendered a subject may be, it is of little value as a medical illustration *if it does not serve to make clear some medical point.*" Dr. Netter's planning, conception, point of view, and approach are what inform his paintings and what makes them so intellectually valuable.

Frank H. Netter, M.D., physician and artist, died in 1991.

About the Authors

John T. Hansen, Ph.D., is Professor and Associate Chair for Education in Neurobiology and Anatomy, Associate Dean for Admissions, and Director of Curriculum Development in the Offices of Medical Education at the University of Rochester School of Medicine and Dentistry. Dr. Hansen served as Chair of the Department of Neurobiology and Anatomy before becoming Associate Dean. Dr. Hansen is the recipient of numerous teaching awards from students at three different medical schools. In 1999, he was the recipient of The Alpha Omega Alpha Robert J. Glaser Distinguished Teacher Award given annually by the Association of American Medical Colleges to nationally recognized medical educators. Dr. Hansen's investigative career encompasses research of the peripheral chemoreceptor system, paraneurons, and neural plasticity and inflammation. He is author of *Essential Anatomy Dissector* and editor on the CD-ROM *Netter Presenter Human Anatomy Collection.*

Bruce M. Koeppen, M.D., Ph.D., is Professor of Medicine and Physiology and Dean for Academic Affairs and Education at the University of Connecticut School of Medicine. Dr. Koeppen is the recipient of numerous teaching awards from the students at the University of Connecticut Schools of Medicine and Dental Medicine. In 1995, he was the recipient of the Arthur C. Guyton Teaching Award from the American Society of Physiology, and he was the 1998 recipient of The Alpha Omega Alpha Robert J. Glaser Distinguished Teacher Award given annually by the Association of American Medical Colleges to nationally recognized medical educators. Dr. Koeppen's investigative career encompasses research in renal physiology and, more recently, medical education. He is coauthor of the textbook *Renal Physiology,* contributing author to *Principles of Physiology,* and contributing author and editor of *Berne and Levy's Textbook of Physiology.*

Acknowledgments

Preparing this *Atlas* has been a true joy. Like any project of this kind, a number of people have helped make it a reality. First, we are indebted to all of our former students who have inspired and challenged us to be better teachers. This *Atlas* is for them and for future students of physiology who, like us, will grapple with the complexities of a novel discipline and yearn for a better view of the larger picture.

Thanks and appreciation also to our colleagues and reviewers who provided encouragement and constructive comments that clarified many aspects of this *Atlas*. Especially, we wish to acknowledge Drs. Dan Henry, Russell Hilf, Ralph Józefowicz, Bruce Stanton, John West, and David Yule. A special thanks to Ms. Edith Müller and Professor Heini Murer, Sekretariat of the Universität Zürich Physiologisches Institut for sharing their hospitality and allowing one of us (BK) to spend the summer at their institution while preparing the first draft of this book. We hope that at least some of each of these colleague's abiding love of physiology is embodied in the beautiful artwork that illustrates this *Atlas*. Like us, they believe that structure and function are a continuum and that the beauty and awe of human physiology can be captured visually, from the organ to the cell and molecular level.

At Icon Learning Systems, it has been a distinct pleasure working with a staff of dedicated and professional people who made this novel dream a published reality. We sincerely appreciate and gratefully acknowledge the efforts of Jennifer Surich, Managing Editor and the person most responsible for keeping us "on task and focused"; Michelle Jahn, Art Production Manager; Jim O'Keeffe, Print Production Manager; Joan Caldwell, Marketing Manager; and Greg Otis, Vice President and Editorial Director.

We would also like to thank Suzanne Kastner, Project Manager at Graphic World, who was responsible for coordinating the composition of the textbook and art.

A very special thank you and debt of gratitude is reserved for Paul Kelly, Executive Editor at Icon Learning Systems, who was the first to believe in our philosophy of the "30,000-foot view" as a key to learning any complex discipline. Paul listened patiently, asked the right questions, and embraced the idea that physiology also is a visual science that can come alive for students who yearn to see.

Special thanks also to Jim Perkins, John Craig, M.D., and Carlos Machado, M.D., for their beautiful artistic renderings of physiological concepts that nicely complement and update the legendary Netter illustrations. Jim, John, and Carlos, in true Netter parlance, "clarified" rather than "intimidated," and their professionalism and expertise made our job enjoyable and significantly easier.

Finally, we remain indebted to Frank H. Netter, M.D., whose unique perspective and understanding of structure-function relationships informed our own graduate and medical learning, and provided the creative impetus for this *Atlas*. Generations of biomedical professionals owe a debt of gratitude to Dr. Netter's artwork, and we feel privileged and humbled to carry forth his legacy to future generations.

To all these individuals, and others—"Thank you."

John T. Hansen, Ph.D.
Bruce M. Koeppen, M.D., Ph.D.

Contents

Chapter 1 Cell Physiology

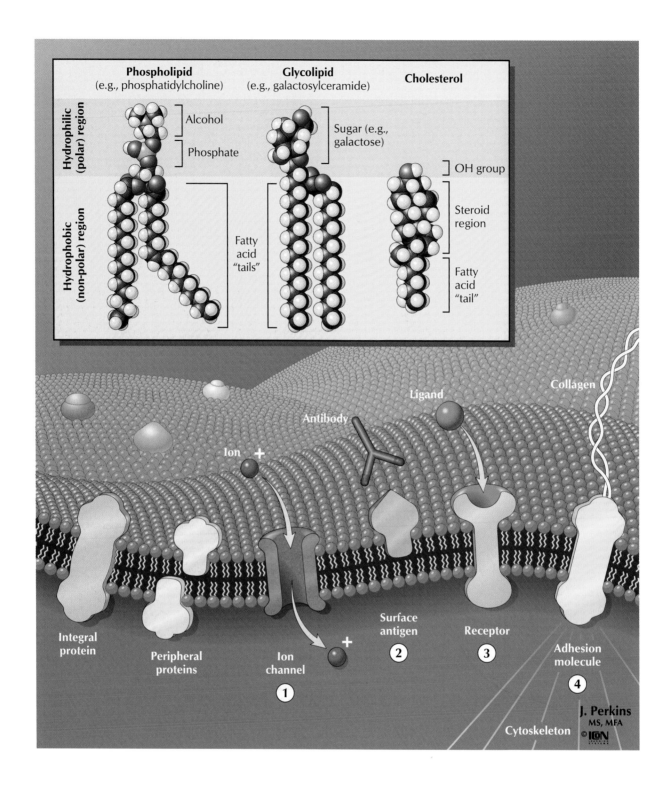

FIGURE 1.1   EUKARYOTIC CELL PLASMA MEMBRANE STRUCTURE

The plasma membrane of eukaryotic cells consists of a lipid bilayer and integral and peripheral proteins. Phospholipids are the major component of the bilayer. Cholesterol is also present in the bilayer and helps maintain appropriate membrane fluidity. Glycolipid helps anchor peripheral proteins to the membrane. The membrane-associated proteins serve many important cellular functions, including (1) transport of biologically important substances into and out of the cell (e.g., ion channels), (2) cell recognition (e.g., surface antigens), (3) cell-to-cell communication (e.g., neurotransmitter and hormone receptors), and (4) tissue organization (e.g., adhesion molecules).

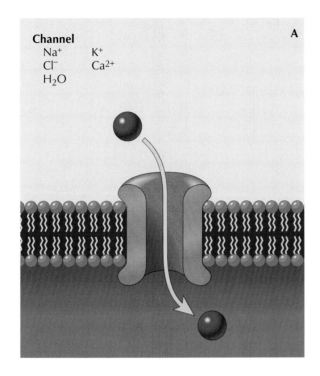

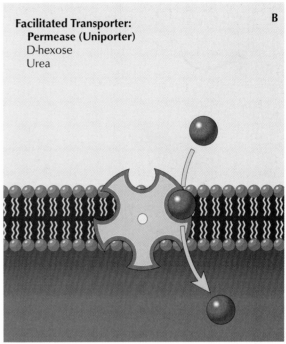

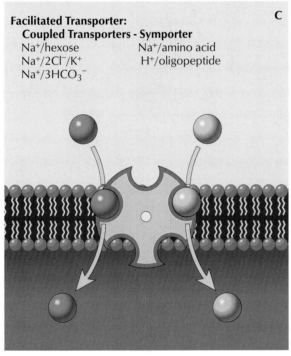

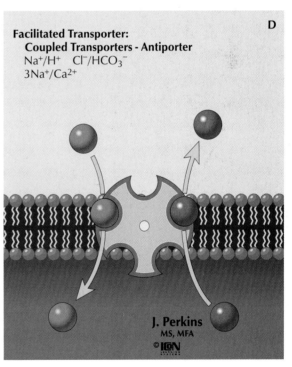

FIGURE 1.2   MEMBRANE TRANSPORT: I

Transporters are a diverse group of integral membrane proteins that move biologically important substances into and out of the cell. Transporters confer specificity to the movement of substances across the membrane and allow this movement to be regulated by the cell. **A. Facilitated diffusion via ion channels:** Integral membrane proteins span the membrane and provide an aqueous pore by which ions (e.g., Na⁺, K⁺, Cl⁻, and Ca²⁺) can cross the membrane. **B–D. Facilitated diffusion via carrier proteins:** Sugars and amino acids are important to the cell and can cross the membrane by binding with an integral membrane protein carrier, which then releases the solute on the opposite side.

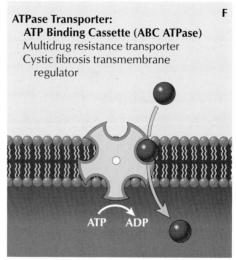

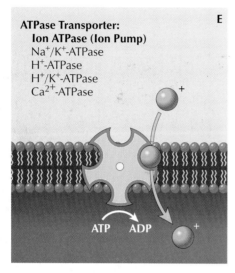

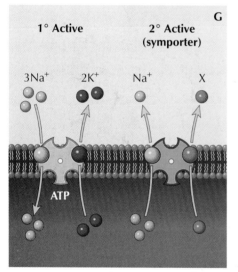

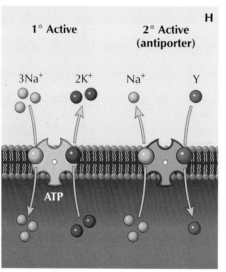

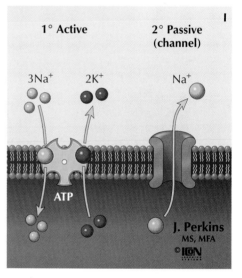

FIGURE 1.2   MEMBRANE TRANSPORT: I—CONT'D

E–F. Transport via ATPase transporters: Ions can be transported across the membrane driven by the energy in ATP (ion pumps). Larger molecules (e.g., drugs) can also be transported by integral membrane proteins that also utilize ATP (ABC ATPase). **G–I. Primary active phransport:** Direct use of metabolic energy to transport ions against a concentration or electrical potential gradient (e.g., ion pumps, such as the Na$^+$-K$^+$-ATPase). **G–I. Secondary active**

transport: Movement of solutes against a concentration or electrical potential gradient, but not directly coupled to metabolic energy. The energy for transport is derived from coupling to the movement of another solute. **Simple diffusion:** Lipid-soluble molecules and gases (e.g., O_2, CO_2) can diffuse through the lipid portion of the membrane driven by a concentration gradient (not depicted).

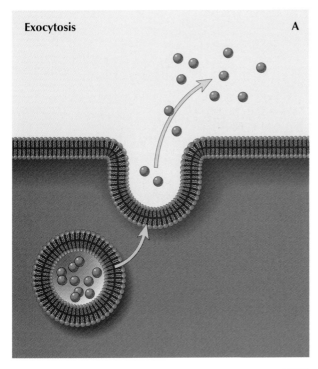

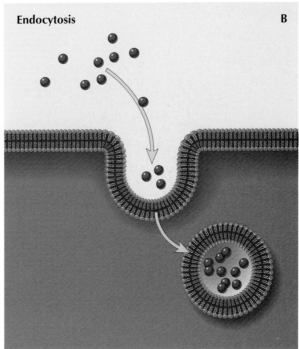

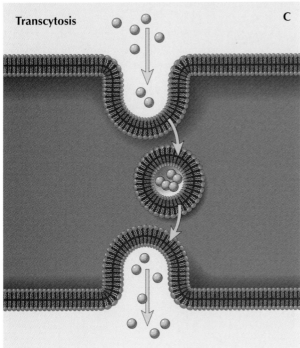

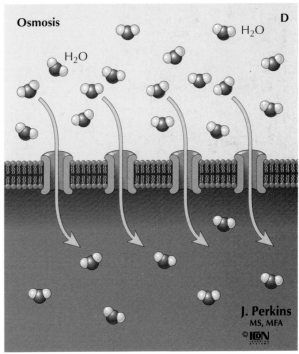

FIGURE 1.3   MEMBRANE TRANSPORT: II

Substances can be brought into, or expelled from, the cell by membrane-bound vesicles. This mode of transport requires ATP and may be either nonspecific or highly specific as a result of the presence of receptor molecules in the membrane of the vesicles. **A. Exocytosis:** Extrusion from the cell involving fusion of an intracellular vesicle with the cell membrane. **B. Endocytosis:** The opposite of exocytosis (also called phagocytosis, pinocytosis).

C. Transcytosis: Endothelial cells of capillaries and epithelial cells of the intestine shuttle material across the cell by a process of endocytosis and exocytosis, called transcytosis. **D. Osmosis:** Water moves across cell membranes by the process of osmosis. Water movement is always passive and driven through water channels (aquaporins) by an osmotic pressure gradient.

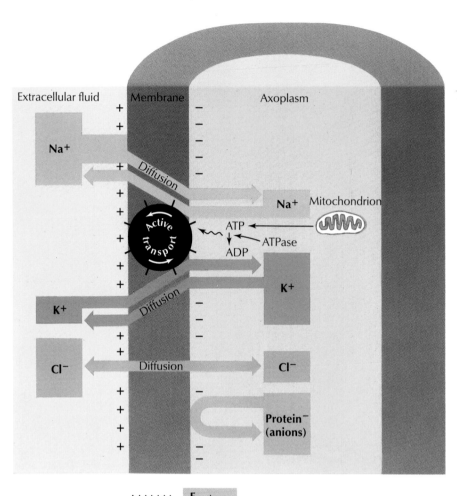

$$E_K = 61 \log \frac{[K^+ \text{ outside}]}{K^+ \text{ inside}}$$

$$E_{Na} = 61 \log \frac{[Na^+ \text{ outside}]}{Na^+ \text{ inside}}$$

$$E_{Cl} = -61 \log \frac{[Cl^- \text{ outside}]}{Cl^- \text{ inside}}$$

FIGURE 1.4 RESTING MEMBRANE POTENTIAL

Ions are distributed across the cell membrane in an asymmetric manner. Extracellular fluid has high concentrations of Na^+ (145 mEq/L) and Cl^- (105 mEq/L) and a low concentration of K^+ (3.5 mEq/L). Conversely, the intracellular concentrations of Na^+ (15 mEq/L) and Cl^- (8 mEq/L) are low, whereas that of K^+ (130 mEq/L) is high. The distribution of ions across the cell membrane depends on the activity of the Na^+-K^+-ATPase. By its activity, Na^+ is actively pumped out of the cell

and K^+ is actively pumped into the cell. Some of the K^+ leaks out of the cell through K^+-selective channels. It is this leak of K^+ out of the cell that is largely responsible for establishing the resting membrane potential. A convenient way to model the generation of the resting membrane potential is by means of an equivalent circuit diagram. In such a diagram the energy in the ion gradients is expressed in millivolts (mV). These values are calculated using the Nernst equation.

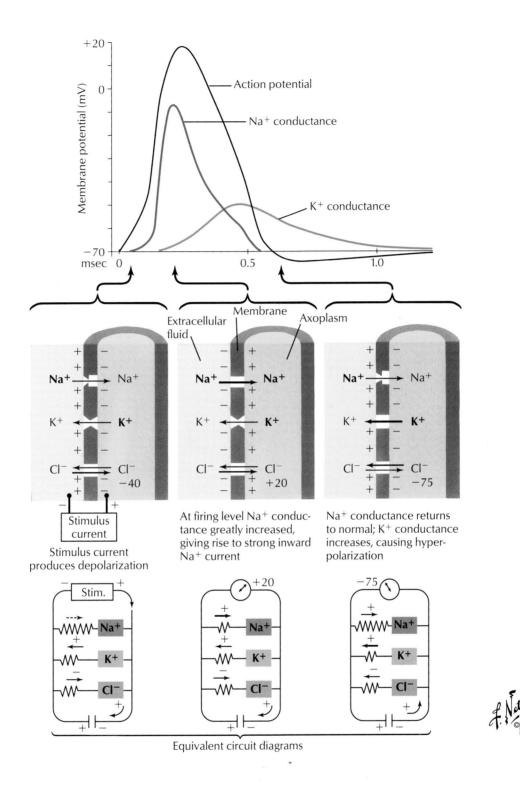

FIGURE 1.5　ACTION POTENTIAL

The generation and conduction of action potentials is critically important for the function of excitable tissues (e.g., neurons, muscle). The process has been extensively studied in the axon of neurons. With membrane depolarization (e.g., as a result of a neurotransmitter acting at a synapse), there is a local depolarization of the resting membrane potential. If this is of a sufficient magnitude (threshold voltage), it causes voltage-sensitive Na$^+$ channels to open and the action potential is initiated. These Na$^+$ channels rapidly close, and the associated membrane depolarization opens K$^+$ selective channels. This increased K$^+$ conductance of the membrane repolarizes the cell to its resting potential.

A. Myelinated fibers

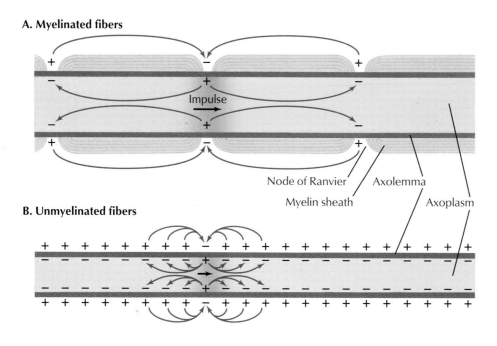

Node of Ranvier　　Axolemma

Myelin sheath　　　Axoplasm

B. Unmyelinated fibers

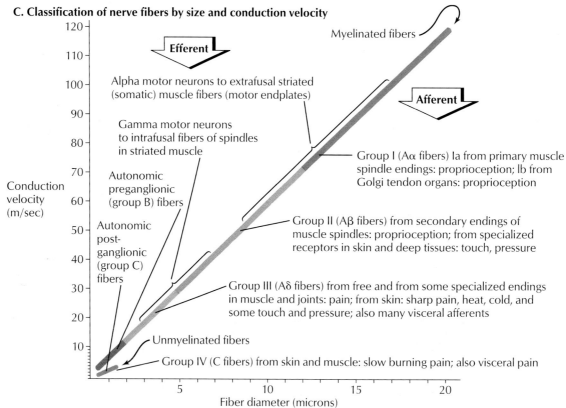

C. Classification of nerve fibers by size and conduction velocity

Myelinated fibers

Efferent

Afferent

Alpha motor neurons to extrafusal striated (somatic) muscle fibers (motor endplates)

Gamma motor neurons to intrafusal fibers of spindles in striated muscle

Autonomic preganglionic (group B) fibers

Autonomic post-ganglionic (group C) fibers

Conduction velocity (m/sec)

Group I (Aα fibers) Ia from primary muscle spindle endings: proprioception; Ib from Golgi tendon organs: proprioception

Group II (Aβ fibers) from secondary endings of muscle spindles: proprioception; from specialized receptors in skin and deep tissues: touch, pressure

Group III (Aδ fibers) from free and from some specialized endings in muscle and joints: pain; from skin: sharp pain, heat, cold, and some touch and pressure; also many visceral afferents

Unmyelinated fibers

Group IV (C fibers) from skin and muscle: slow burning pain; also visceral pain

Fiber diameter (microns)

FIGURE 1.6　CONDUCTION VELOCITY

The action potential travels down the axon by depolarizing adjacent membrane sections (panel B). The speed of propagation increases with larger axonal diameter and in the presence of a myelin sheath (panel C). In myelinated axons the action potential is transmitted node to node, a process called saltatory conduction (panel A).

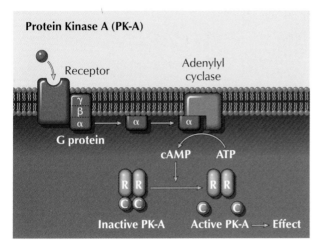

Protein Kinase A (PK-A)

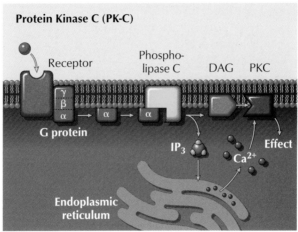

Protein Kinase C (PK-C)

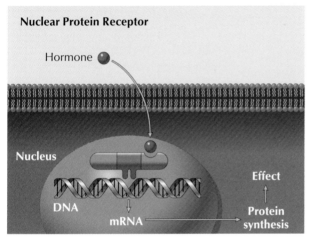

Nuclear Protein Receptor

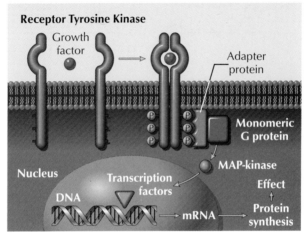

Receptor Tyrosine Kinase

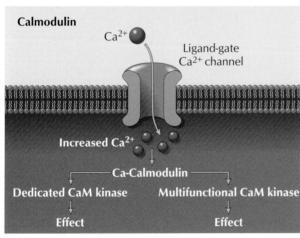

Calmodulin

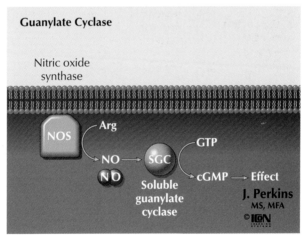

Guanylate Cyclase

J. Perkins
MS, MFA
© ICON

FIGURE 1.7   SIGNAL TRANSDUCTION PATHWAYS: I

Communication between cells involves receptors (often integral membrane proteins) and a coupling of the receptor to effector proteins in the cell. These signal transduction pathways are important for regulating the function of cells. Responses of the cell (i.e., effect) include such things as alteration in enzyme function, synthesis of cellular proteins, secretion of proteins, and cell growth and division. Some of the more common signal transduction pathways are depicted here in simplified form. (*Abbreviations: Arg,* Arginine; *CaM kinase,* Ca^{2+}/calmodulin-dependent protein kinase; *DAG,* diacylglycerol; *IP$_3$,* inositol 1,4,5-trisphosphate; *MAP-kinase,* mitogen-activated protein kinase; *NO,* nitric oxide.)

CHART 1.1 G PROTEINS

Heterotrimeric G proteins couple receptors to a number of different cellular effector proteins (e.g., enzymes, ion channels). Some of the known G proteins are summarized.

G Protein	Activated by Receptors for	Effectors	Signaling Pathways
G_s	Epinephrine, norepinephrine, histamine, glucagon, ACTH, luteinizing hormone, follicle-stimulating hormone, thyroid-stimulating hormone, others	Adenylyl cyclase Ca^{2+} channels	↑ Cyclic AMP ↑ Ca^{2+} influx
G_{olf}	Odorants	Adenylyl cyclase	↑ AMP (olfaction)
G_{r1} (rods)	Photons	Cyclic GMP phosphodiesterase	↓ Cyclic GMP (vision)
G_{r2} (cones)	Photons	Cyclic GMP phosphodiesterase	↓ Cyclic GMP (color vision)
G_{i1}, G_{i2}, G_{i3}	Norepinephrine, prostaglandins, opiates, angiotensin, many peptides	Adenylyl cyclase Phospholipase C Phospholipase A$_2$ K$^+$ channels	↓ Cyclic AMP ↑ Inositol 1,4,5-trisphosphate, diacylglycerol, Ca^{2+} Membrane polarization
G_q	Acetylcholine, epinephrine	Phospholipase Cβ	↑ Inositol 1,4,5-trisphosphate, diacylglycerol, Ca^{2+}

ACTH, Adrenocorticotropic hormone.

Note: There is more than one isoform of each class of a subunit. More than 20 distinct α subunits have been identified.

CHART 1.2 SIGNAL TRANSDUCTION PATHWAYS

Summary of some hormones, neurotransmitters and drugs, and the signal transduction pathways involved in their actions on cells.

Adenylyl Cyclase (cAMP)	Phospholipase C (IP$_3$ – Ca^{2+})	Cytoplasmic/Nuclear Receptor	Tyrosine Kinase	Guanylate Cyclase (cGMP)
ACTH	GnRH*	Cortisol	Insulin	ANP
LH	TRH*	Estradiol	IGFs	Nitric oxide
FSH	GHRH*	Progesterone	GH	
ADH (V$_2$ receptor)	CRH*	Testosterone		
PTH	Angiotensin II	Aldosterone		
Calcitonin	ADH (V$_1$ receptor)	Calcitriol		
Glucagon	oxytocin	Thyroid hormones		
β-Adrenergic agonists	α-Adrenergic agonists			

*Also increase intracellular cAMP.

ACTH, Adrenocorticotropic hormone; *ADH,* antidiuretic hormone (vasopressin); *ANP,* atrial natriuretic peptide; *CRH,* corticotropin-releasing hormone; *FSH,* follicle-stimulating hormone; *GH,* growth hormone; *GHRH,* growth hormone–releasing hormone; *GnRH,* gonadotropin-releasing hormone; *IGF,* insulin-like growth factor; *LH,* luteinizing hormone; *PTH,* parathyroid hormone; *TRH,* thyrotropin-releasing hormone.

Chapter 2 Neurophysiology

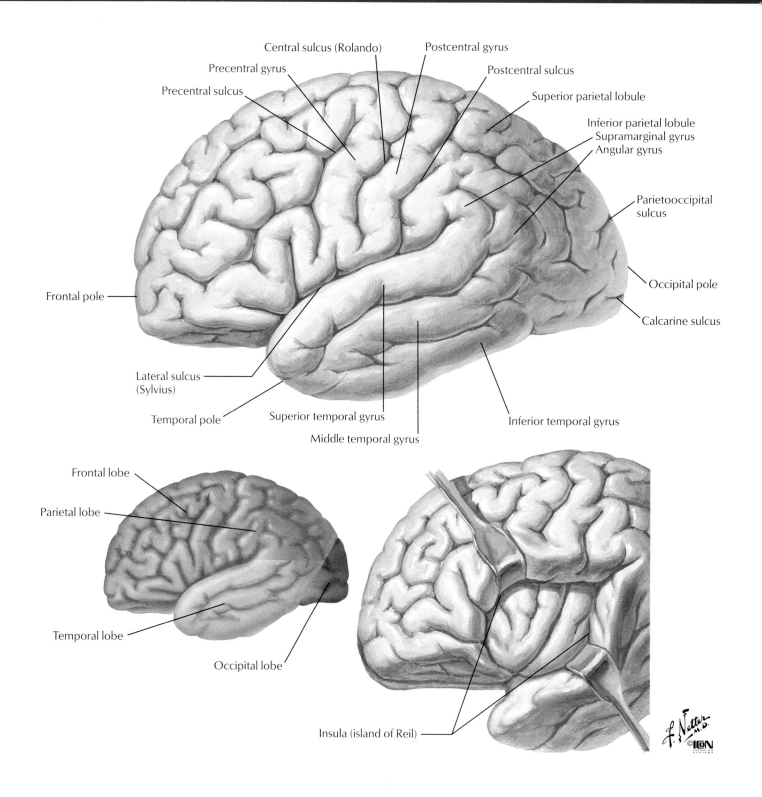

FIGURE 2.1   ORGANIZATION OF THE BRAIN: CEREBRUM

The cerebral cortex represents the highest center for sensory and motor processing. In general, the frontal lobe processes motor, visual, speech, and personality modalities. The parietal lobe processes sensory information; the temporal lobe, auditory and memory modalities; and the occipital lobe, vision. The cerebellum coordinates smooth motor activities and processes muscle position. The brainstem (medulla, pons, midbrain) conveys motor and sensory information and mediates important autonomic functions. The spinal cord receives sensory input from the body and conveys somatic and autonomic motor information to peripheral targets (muscles, viscera).

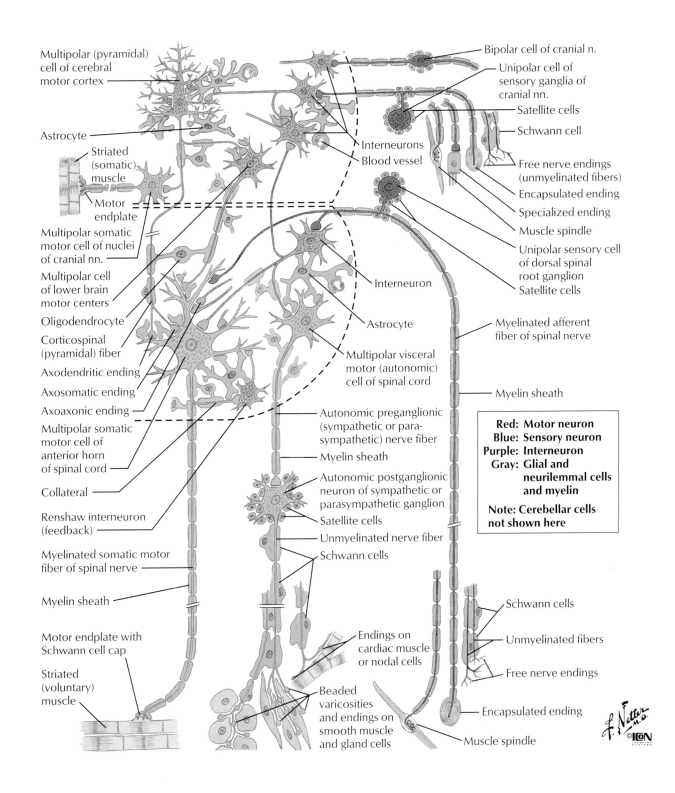

FIGURE 2.2   ORGANIZATION OF THE BRAIN: CELL TYPES

Neurons form the functional cellular units responsible for communication, and throughout the nervous system, they are characterized by their distinctive size and shapes (e.g., bipolar, unipolar, multipolar). Supporting cells include the neuroglia (e.g., astrocytes, oligodendrocytes), satellite cells, and other specialized cells that optimize neuronal function, provide maintenance functions, or protect the nervous system.

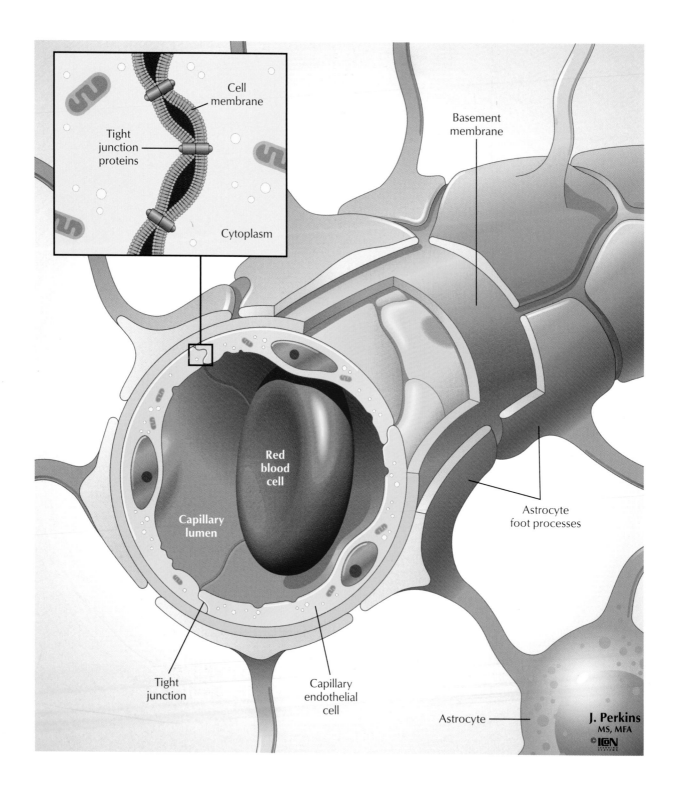

Figure 2.3 Blood-Brain Barrier

The blood-brain barrier (BBB) is the cellular interface between the blood and the central nervous system (CNS; brain and spinal cord). It serves to maintain the interstitial fluid environment to ensure optimal functionality of the neurons. This barrier consists of the capillary endothelial cells with an elaborate network of tight junctions and astrocytic foot processes that abut the endothelium and its basement membrane. The movement of large molecules and other substances (including many drugs) from the blood to the interstitial space of the CNS is restricted by the BBB. CNS endothelial cells also exhibit a low level of pinocytotic activity across the cell, so specific carrier systems for the transport of essential substrates of energy and amino acid metabolism are characteristic of these cells. The astrocytes help transfer important metabolites from the blood to the neurons and also remove excess K^+ and neurotransmitters from the interstitial fluid.

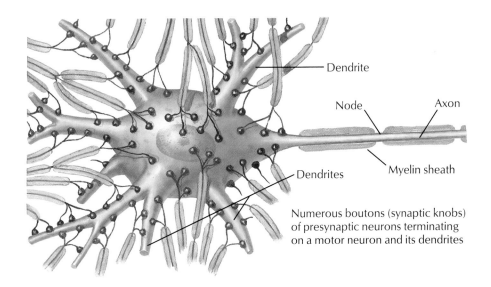

Dendrite

Node — Axon

Myelin sheath

Dendrites

Numerous boutons (synaptic knobs) of presynaptic neurons terminating on a motor neuron and its dendrites

Enlarged section of bouton

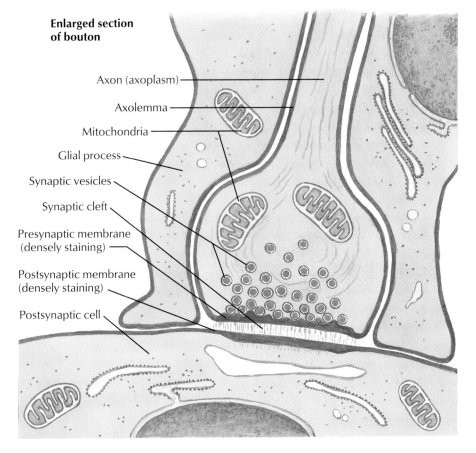

Axon (axoplasm)

Axolemma

Mitochondria

Glial process

Synaptic vesicles

Synaptic cleft

Presynaptic membrane (densely staining)

Postsynaptic membrane (densely staining)

Postsynaptic cell

FIGURE 2.4   MORPHOLOGY OF SYNAPSES

Neurons communicate with each other and with effector targets at specialized regions called synapses. The top figure shows a typical motor neuron that receives numerous synaptic contacts on its cell body and associated dendrites. Incoming axons lose their myelin sheaths, exhibit extensive branching, and terminate as synaptic boutons (synaptic terminals or knobs) on the motor neuron. The lower figure shows an enlargement of one such synaptic bouton. Chemical neurotransmitters are contained in synaptic vesicles, which can fuse with the presynaptic membrane, release the transmitters into the synaptic cleft, and then bind to receptors situated in the postsynaptic membrane. This synaptic transmission results in excitatory, inhibitory, or modulatory effects on the target cell.

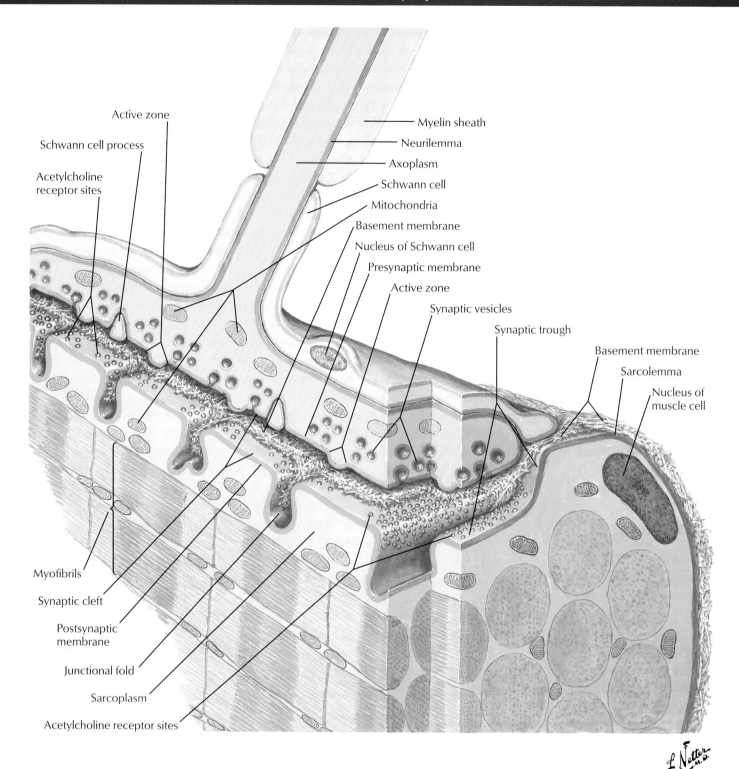

Active zone
Schwann cell process
Acetylcholine receptor sites
Myelin sheath
Neurilemma
Axoplasm
Schwann cell
Mitochondria
Basement membrane
Nucleus of Schwann cell
Presynaptic membrane
Active zone
Synaptic vesicles
Synaptic trough
Basement membrane
Sarcolemma
Nucleus of muscle cell
Myofibrils
Synaptic cleft
Postsynaptic membrane
Junctional fold
Sarcoplasm
Acetylcholine receptor sites

FIGURE 2.5   STRUCTURE OF THE NEUROMUSCULAR JUNCTION

Motor axons that synapse on skeletal muscle form expanded terminals called neuromuscular junctions (motor endplates). The motor axon loses its myelin sheath and expands into a Schwann cell–invested synaptic terminal that resides within a trough in the muscle fiber. Acetylcholine-containing synaptic vesicles accumulate adjacent to the presynaptic membrane and, when appropriately stimulated, release their neurotransmitter into the synaptic cleft. The transmitter then binds to receptors that mediate depolarization of the muscle sarcolemma and initiate a muscle action potential. A single muscle fiber has only one neuromuscular junction, but a motor axon can innervate multiple muscle fibers.

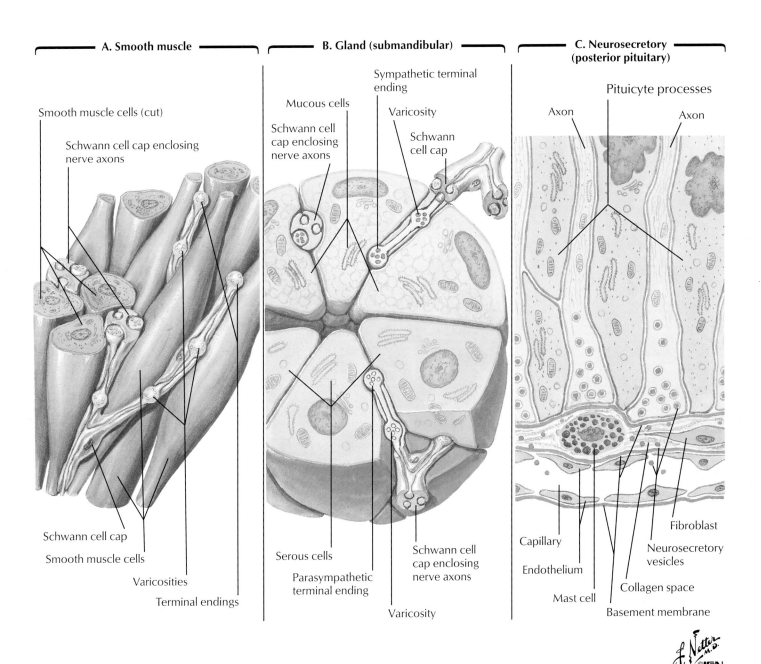

A. Smooth muscle

Smooth muscle cells (cut)

Schwann cell cap enclosing nerve axons

Schwann cell cap

Smooth muscle cells

Varicosities

Terminal endings

B. Gland (submandibular)

Sympathetic terminal ending

Mucous cells

Varicosity

Schwann cell cap enclosing nerve axons

Schwann cell cap

Serous cells

Parasympathetic terminal ending

Schwann cell cap enclosing nerve axons

Varicosity

C. Neurosecretory (posterior pituitary)

Pituicyte processes

Axon

Axon

Fibroblast

Neurosecretory vesicles

Capillary

Endothelium

Collagen space

Mast cell

Basement membrane

FIGURE 2.6 VISCERAL EFFERENT ENDINGS

Neuronal efferent endings on smooth muscle (A) and glands (B and C) exhibit unique endings unlike the presynaptic and postsynaptic terminals observed in neuronal and neuromuscular junction synapses. Rather, neurotransmitter substances are released into interstitial spaces (A and B) or into the bloodstream (C, neu-rosecretion) from expanded nerve terminal endings. This arrangement allows for the stimulation of numerous target cells over a wide area. Not all smooth muscle cells are innervated. They are connected to adjacent cells by gap junctions and can therefore contract together with the innervated cells.

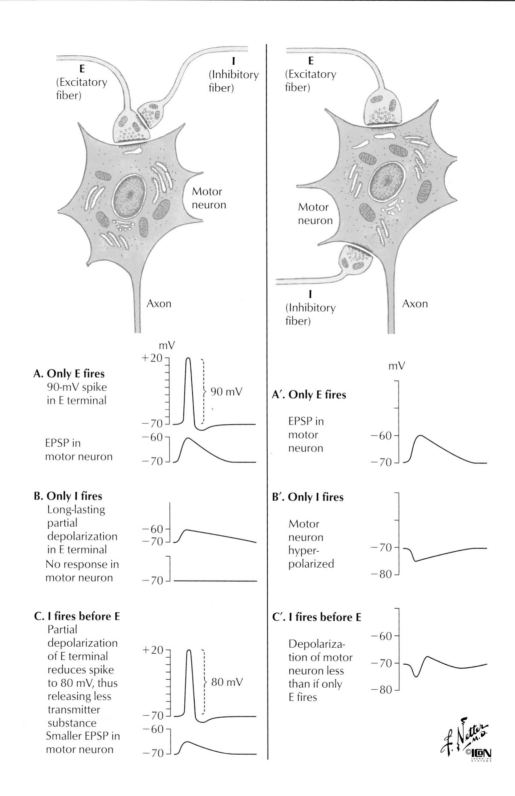

FIGURE 2.7 SYNAPTIC INHIBITORY MECHANISMS

Inhibitory synapses modulate neuronal activity. Illustrated here is presynaptic inhibition (left panel) and postsynaptic inhibition (right panel) at a motor neuron.

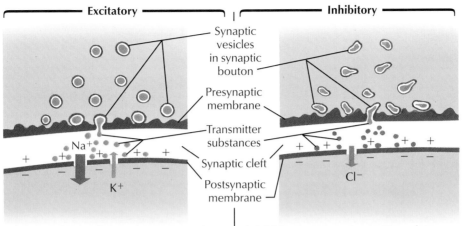

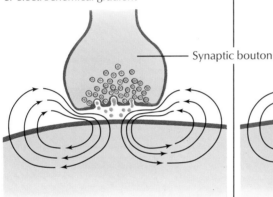

When impulse reaches excitatory synaptic bouton, it causes release of a transmitter substance into synaptic cleft. This increases permeability of postsynaptic membrane to Na⁺ and K⁺. More Na⁺ moves into postsynaptic cell than K⁺ moves out, due to greater electrochemical gradient

At inhibitory synapse, transmitter substance released by an impulse increases permeability of the postsynaptic membrane to Cl⁻. K⁺ moves out of post-synaptic cell but no net flow of Cl⁻ occurs at resting membrane potential

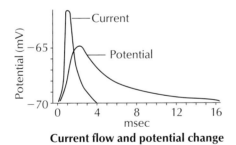

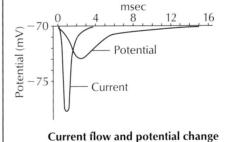

Resultant net ionic current flow is in a direction that tends to depolarize postsynaptic cell. If depolarization reaches firing threshold, an impulse is generated in postsynaptic cell

Resultant ionic current flow is in direction that tends to hyperpolarize postsynaptic cell. This makes depolarization by excitatory synapses more difficult—more depolarization is required to reach threshold

Current flow and potential change

Current flow and potential change

FIGURE 2.8   CHEMICAL SYNAPTIC TRANSMISSION

Chemical synaptic transmission between neurons may be excitatory or inhibitory. During excitation (left column), a net increase in the inward flow of Na⁺ compared with the outward flow of K⁺ results in a depolarizing potential change (excitatory postsynaptic potential [EPSP]) that drives the postsynaptic cell closer to its threshold for an action potential. During inhibition (right column), the opening of K⁺ and Cl⁻ channels drives the membrane potential away from threshold (hyperpolarization) and decreases the probability that the neuron will reach threshold (inhibitory postsynaptic potential [IPSP]) for an action potential.

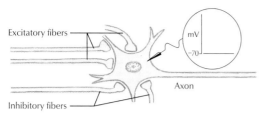

A. Resting state: motor nerve cell shown with synaptic boutons of excitatory and inhibitory nerve fibers ending close to it

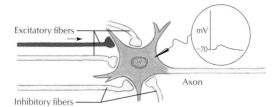

B. Partial depolarization: impulse from one excitatory fiber has caused partial (below firing threshold) depolarization of motor neuron

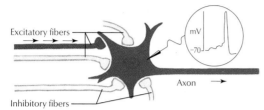

C. Temporal excitatory summation: a series of impulses in one excitatory fiber together produce a suprathreshold depolarization that triggers an action potential

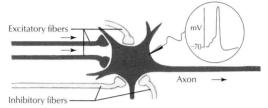

D. Spatial excitatory summation: impulses in two excitatory fibers cause two synaptic depolarizations that together reach firing threshold triggering an action potential

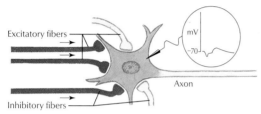

E. Spatial excitatory summation with inhibition: impulses from two excitatory fibers reach motor neuron but impulses from inhibitory fiber prevent depolarization from reaching threshold

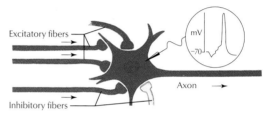

E. (continued): motor neuron now receives additional excitatory impulses and reaches firing threshold despite a simultaneous inhibitory impulse; additional inhibitory impulses might still prevent firing

CHART 2.1   SUMMARY OF SOME NEUROTRANSMITTERS AND WHERE WITHIN THE CENTRAL AND PERIPHERAL NERVOUS SYSTEM THEY ARE FOUND

Transmitter	Location	Transmitter	Location
Acetylcholine	Neuromuscular junction, autonomic endings and ganglia, CNS	Gas Nitric oxide	CNS, GI tract

Biogenic amines
    Norepinephrine
    Dopamine
    Serotonin
	
	Sympathetic endings, CNS
	CNS
	CNS, GI tract
		Peptides
		    β-Endorphins
		    Enkephalins
		    Antidiuretic
		    hormone
			
			CNS, GI tract
			CNS
			CNS (hypothalamus/posterior
			pituitary)

Amino acids
    γ-Aminobutyric
    acid (GABA)
    Glutamate
	
	CNS
	
	CNS
		Pituitary-releasing
		    hormones
		    Somatostatin
		    Neuropeptide Y
		    Vasoactive
		    intestinal peptide
			CNS (hypothalamus/anterior
			pituitary)
			CNS, GI tract
			CNS
			
			CNS, GI tract

Purines
    Adenosine
    Adenosine
    triphosphate (ATP)
	
	CNS
	CNS		

CNS, Central nervous system; *GI,* gastrointestinal.

FIGURE 2.9   TEMPORAL AND SPATIAL SUMMATION

Neurons receive multiple excitatory and inhibitory inputs. Temporal summation occurs when a series of subthreshold impulses in one excitatory fiber produces an action potential in the postsynaptic cell (panel C). Spatial summation occurs when subthreshold impulses from two or more different fibers trigger an action poten-tial (panel D). Both temporal and spatial summation can be modulated by simultaneous inhibitory input (panel E). Inhibitory and excitatory neurons use a wide variety of neurotransmitters, some of which are summarized here.

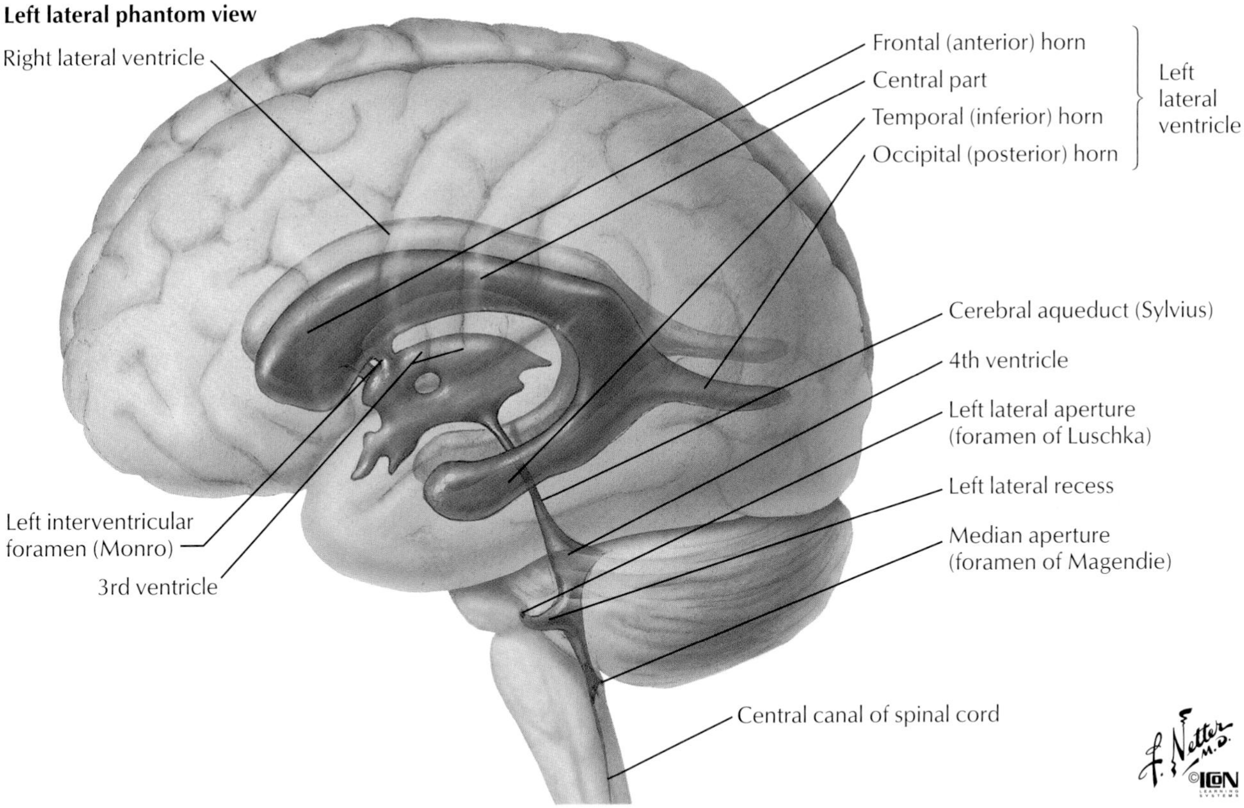
Left lateral phantom view
Right lateral ventricle
Frontal (anterior) horn
Central part
Temporal (inferior) horn
Occipital (posterior) horn
Left lateral ventricle
Cerebral aqueduct (Sylvius)
4th ventricle
Left lateral aperture (foramen of Luschka)
Left lateral recess
Median aperture (foramen of Magendie)
Left interventricular foramen (Monro)
3rd ventricle
Central canal of spinal cord
F. Netter M.D.
©ICON

CHART 2.2 CSF COMPOSITION

	CSF	Blood Plasma
Na^+ (mEq/L)	140–145	135–147
K^+ (mEq/L)	3	3.5–5.0
Cl^- (mEq/L)	115–120	95–105
HCO_3^- (mEq/L)	20	22–28
Glucose (mg/dL)	50–75	70–110
Protein (g/dL)	0.05–0.07	6.0–7.8
pH	7.3	7.35–7.45

FIGURE 2.10 BRAIN VENTRICLES AND CSF COMPOSITION

CSF circulates through the four brain ventricles (two lateral ventricles and a third and fourth ventricle) and in the subarachnoid space surrounding the brain and spinal cord. The electrolyte composition of the CSF is regulated by the choroid plexus, which secretes the CSF. Importantly, the CSF has a lower [HCO_3^-] than plasma and therefore a lower pH. This allows small changes in blood P_{CO_2} to cause changes in CSF pH, which in turn regulates the rate of respiration (see Chapter 5).

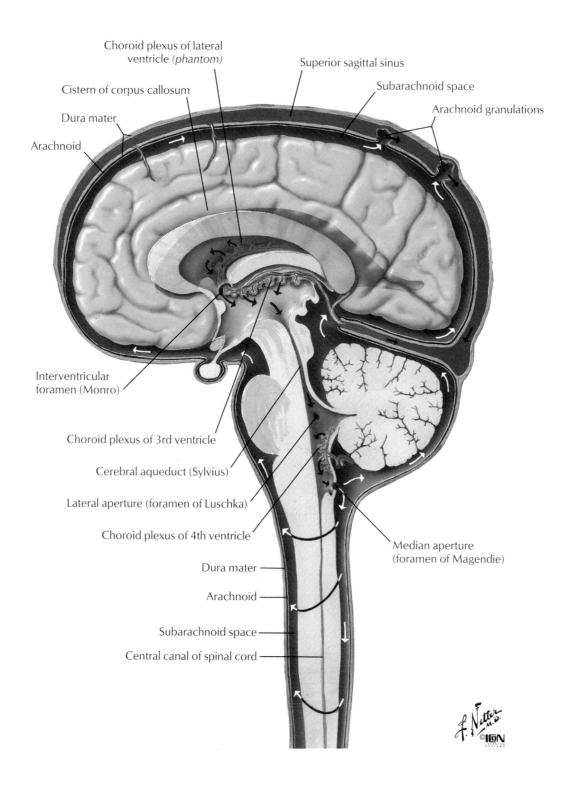

Choroid plexus of lateral ventricle *(phantom)*

Cistern of corpus callosum

Dura mater

Arachnoid

Superior sagittal sinus

Subarachnoid space

Arachnoid granulations

Interventricular foramen (Monro)

Choroid plexus of 3rd ventricle

Cerebral aqueduct (Sylvius)

Lateral aperture (foramen of Luschka)

Choroid plexus of 4th ventricle

Dura mater

Arachnoid

Subarachnoid space

Central canal of spinal cord

Median aperture (foramen of Magendie)

FIGURE 2.11   CIRCULATION OF CEREBROSPINAL FLUID

CSF circulates through the four brain ventricles (two lateral ventricles and a third and fourth ventricle) and in the subarachnoid space surrounding the brain and spinal cord. Most of the CSF is reabsorbed into the venous system through the arachnoid granulations and through the walls of the capillaries of the central nervous system and pia mater.

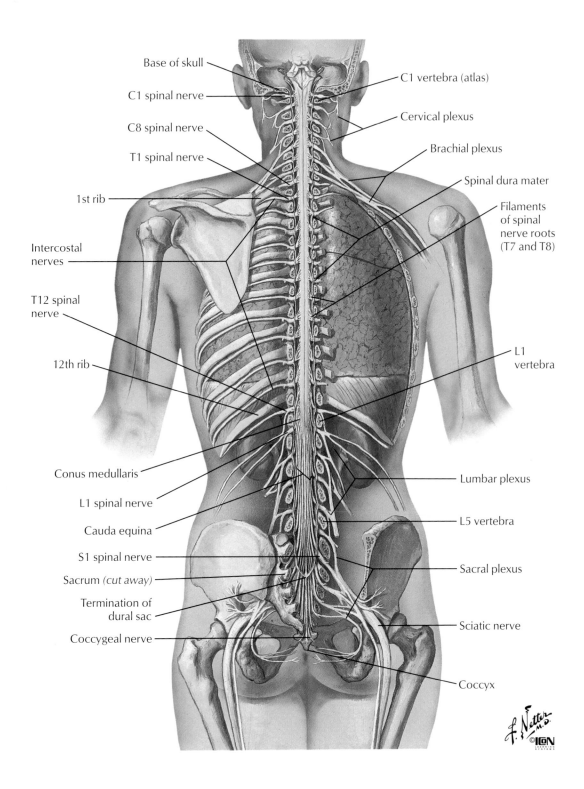

Base of skull

C1 spinal nerve

C8 spinal nerve

T1 spinal nerve

1st rib

Intercostal nerves

T12 spinal nerve

12th rib

Conus medullaris

L1 spinal nerve

Cauda equina

S1 spinal nerve

Sacrum *(cut away)*

Termination of dural sac

Coccygeal nerve

C1 vertebra (atlas)

Cervical plexus

Brachial plexus

Spinal dura mater

Filaments of spinal nerve roots (T7 and T8)

L1 vertebra

Lumbar plexus

L5 vertebra

Sacral plexus

Sciatic nerve

Coccyx

FIGURE 2.12   SPINAL CORD AND VENTRAL RAMI IN SITU

The spinal cord gives rise to 31 pairs of spinal nerves that distribute segmentally to the body. These nerves are organized into plexuses that distribute to the neck (cervical plexus), upper limb (brachial plexus), and pelvis and lower limb (lumbosacral plexus). Motor fibers of these spinal nerves innervate skeletal muscle, and sensory fibers convey information back to the central nervous system from the skin, skeletal muscles, and joints.

23

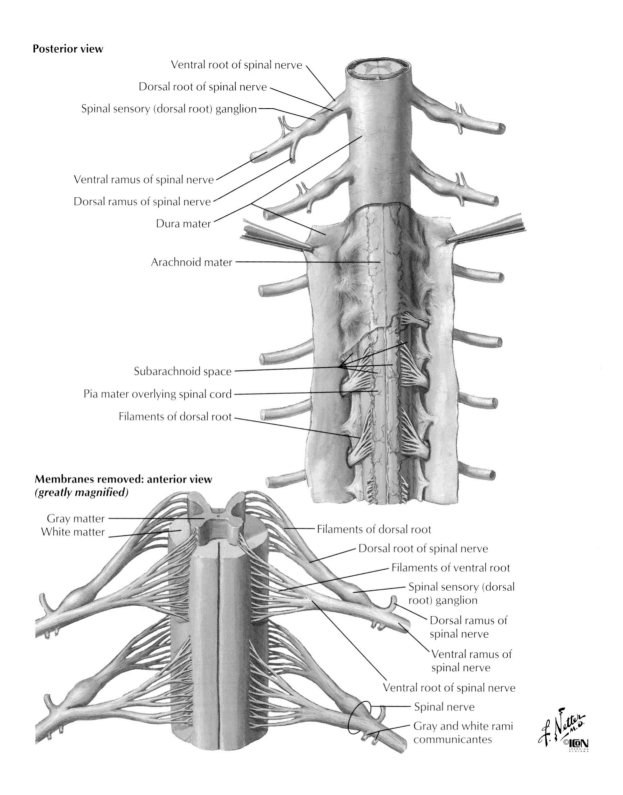

Posterior view

Ventral root of spinal nerve

Dorsal root of spinal nerve

Spinal sensory (dorsal root) ganglion

Ventral ramus of spinal nerve

Dorsal ramus of spinal nerve

Dura mater

Arachnoid mater

Subarachnoid space

Pia mater overlying spinal cord

Filaments of dorsal root

Membranes removed: anterior view
(greatly magnified)

Gray matter

White matter

Filaments of dorsal root

Dorsal root of spinal nerve

Filaments of ventral root

Spinal sensory (dorsal root) ganglion

Dorsal ramus of spinal nerve

Ventral ramus of spinal nerve

Ventral root of spinal nerve

Spinal nerve

Gray and white rami communicantes

FIGURE 2.13   SPINAL MEMBRANES AND NERVE ROOTS

The spinal cord gives rise to 31 pairs of spinal nerves that distribute segmentally to the body. Motor fibers of these spinal nerves innervate skeletal muscle, and sensory fibers convey information back to the central nervous system from the skin, skeletal muscles, and joints.

The spinal cord is ensheathed in three meningeal coverings: the outer, tough dura mater; the arachnoid mater; and the pia mater, which intimately ensheaths the cord itself. CSF bathes the cord and is found in the subarachnoid space.

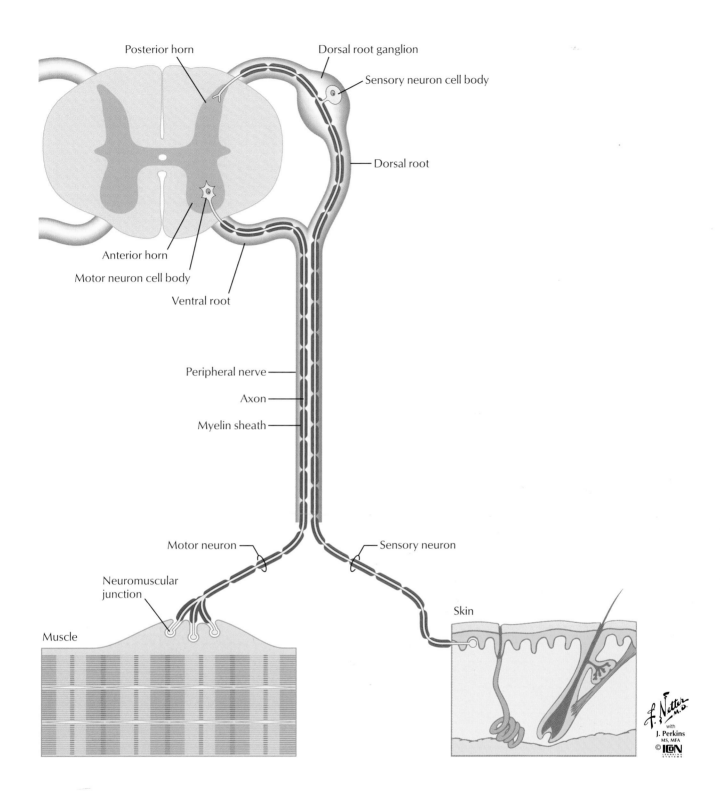

FIGURE 2.14   PERIPHERAL NERVOUS SYSTEM

The peripheral nervous system (PNS) consists of all of the neural elements outside of the CNS (brain and spinal cord) and provides the connections between the CNS and all other body organ systems. The PNS consists of somatic and autonomic components. The somatic component innervates skeletal muscle and skin and is shown here (see Figure 2.15 for the autonomic nervous system). The somatic component of the peripheral nerves contains both motor and sensory axons. Cell bodies of the motor neurons are found in the anterior horn gray matter, whereas the cell bodies of sensory neurons are located in the dorsal root ganglia.

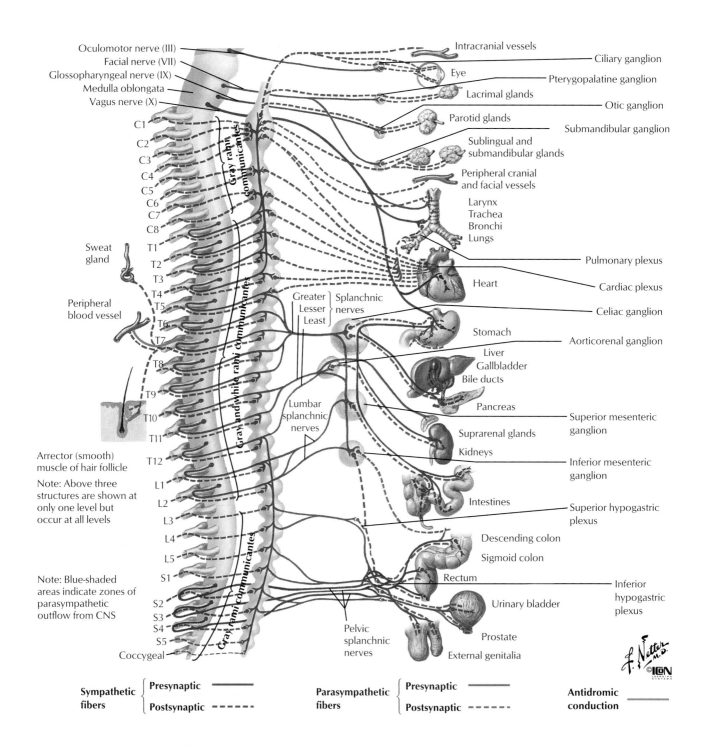

Oculomotor nerve (III)
Facial nerve (VII)
Glossopharyngeal nerve (IX)
Medulla oblongata
Vagus nerve (X)

Intracranial vessels
Ciliary ganglion
Eye
Pterygopalatine ganglion
Lacrimal glands
Otic ganglion
Parotid glands
Submandibular ganglion
Sublingual and submandibular glands

C1
C2
C3
C4
C5
C6
C7
C8

Gray rami communicantes

Peripheral cranial and facial vessels

Larynx
Trachea
Bronchi
Lungs

Sweat gland

T1
T2
T3
T4
T5
T6
T7
T8
T9
T10
T11
T12

Pulmonary plexus
Cardiac plexus
Heart
Celiac ganglion

Peripheral blood vessel

Gray and white rami communicantes

Greater
Lesser
Least

Splanchnic nerves

Stomach
Aorticorenal ganglion
Liver
Gallbladder
Bile ducts

Lumbar splanchnic nerves

Pancreas
Suprarenal glands
Kidneys

Superior mesenteric ganglion
Inferior mesenteric ganglion

Arrector (smooth) muscle of hair follicle

Note: Above three structures are shown at only one level but occur at all levels

L1
L2
L3
L4
L5

Intestines

Superior hypogastric plexus

Descending colon
Sigmoid colon
Rectum

S1
S2
S3
S4
S5
Coccygeal

Gray rami communicantes

Note: Blue-shaded areas indicate zones of parasympathetic outflow from CNS

Urinary bladder
Prostate
External genitalia

Inferior hypogastric plexus

Pelvic splanchnic nerves

| Sympathetic fibers | Presynaptic ——— | Parasympathetic fibers | Presynaptic ——— | Antidromic conduction ——— |
| | Postsynaptic - - - | | Postsynaptic - - - | |

FIGURE 2.15   AUTONOMIC NERVOUS SYSTEM: SCHEMA

The autonomic nervous system is composed of two divisions: the parasympathetic division derived from four of the cranial nerves (CN III, VII, IX, and X) and the S2-S4 sacral spinal cord levels, and the sympathetic division associated with the thoracic and upper lumbar spinal cord levels (T1-L2). The autonomic nervous system is a two-neuron chain, with the preganglionic neuron arising from the central nervous system and synapsing on a postganglionic neuron located in a peripheral autonomic ganglion. Postganglionic axons of the autonomic nervous system innervate smooth muscle, cardiac muscle, and glands. Basically, the sympathetic division mobilizes our body ("fight or flight") while the parasympathetic division regulates digestive and homeostatic functions. Normally, both divisions work in concert to regulate visceral activity (respiration, cardiovascular function, digestion, and associated glandular activity).

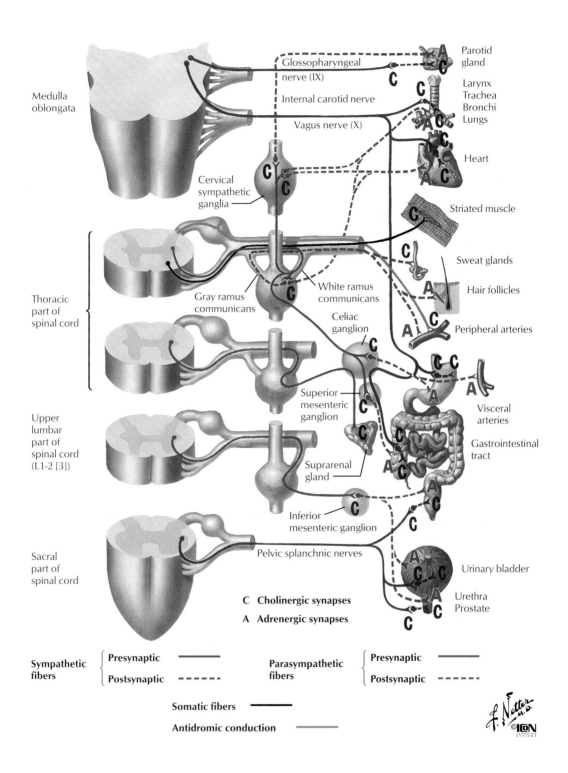

FIGURE 2.16 CHOLINERGIC AND ADRENERGIC SYNAPSES: SCHEMA

The autonomic nervous system (ANS) is a two-neuron chain, with the preganglionic neuron arising from the central nervous system and synapsing on a postganglionic neuron located in a peripheral autonomic ganglion. Acetylcholine is the neurotransmitter in both the sympathetic and parasympathetic ganglia. The parasympathetic division of the ANS releases acetylcholine at its postganglionic synapses and is characterized as having cholinergic (C) effects, whereas the sympathetic division releases predominantly noradren-aline (norepinephrine) at its postganglionic synapses, causing adrenergic (A) effects (except on sweat glands, where acetylcholine is released). Although acetylcholine and noradrenaline are the chief transmitter substances, other neuroactive peptides often are colocalized with them and include such substances as gamma-aminobutyric acid (GABA), substance P, enkephalins, histamine, glutamic acid, neuropeptide Y, and others.

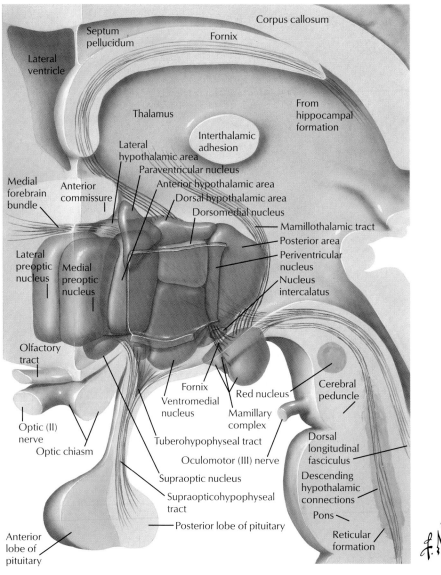

CHART 2.3   MAJOR FUNCTIONS OF THE HYPOTHALAMUS

Hypothalamic Area	Major Functions*
Preoptic and anterior	Heat loss center: cutaneous vasodilation and sweating
Posterior	Heat conservation center: cutaneous vasoconstriction and shivering
Lateral	Feeding center: eating behavior
Ventromedial	Satiety center: inhibits eating behavior
Supraoptic (subfornical organ and organum vasculosum)	ADH and oxytocin secretion (sensation of thirst)
Paraventricular	ADH and oxytocin secretion
Periventricular	Releasing hormones for the anterior pituitary

*Stimulation of the center causes the responses listed.

FIGURE 2.17   SCHEMATIC RECONSTRUCTION OF THE HYPOTHALAMUS

The hypothalamus, part of the diencephalon, controls a number of important homeostatic systems within the body, including temperature regulation, food intake, water intake, many of the endocrine systems (see Chapter 8), motivation, and emotional behavior. It receives inputs from the reticular formation (sleep/wake cycle information), the thalamus (pain), the limbic system (emotion, fear, anger, smell), the medulla oblongata (blood pressure and heart rate), and the optic system, and it integrates these inputs for regulation of the functions listed.

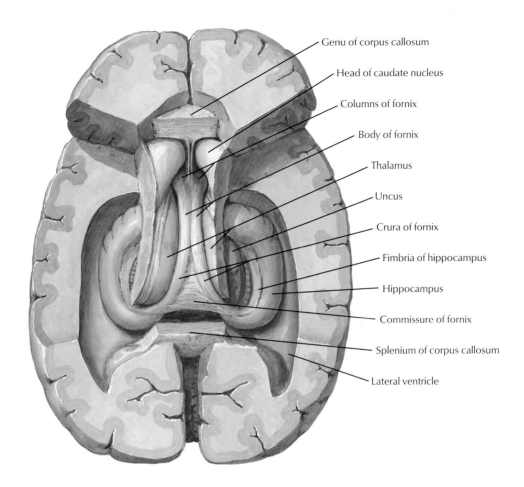

Genu of corpus callosum

Head of caudate nucleus

Columns of fornix

Body of fornix

Thalamus

Uncus

Crura of fornix

Fimbria of hippocampus

Hippocampus

Commissure of fornix

Splenium of corpus callosum

Lateral ventricle

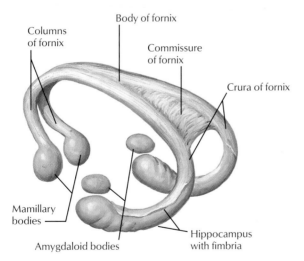

Columns of fornix

Body of fornix

Commissure of fornix

Crura of fornix

Mamillary bodies

Amygdaloid bodies

Hippocampus with fimbria

FIGURE 2.18   HIPPOCAMPUS AND FORNIX

The limbic system includes the hypothalamus and a collection of interconnected structures in the telencephalon (cingulate, parahippocampal, and subcallosal gyri), as well as the amygdala and hippocampal formation. The limbic system functions in linking emotion and motivation (amygdala), learning and memory (hippocampal formation), and sexual behavior (hypothalamus).

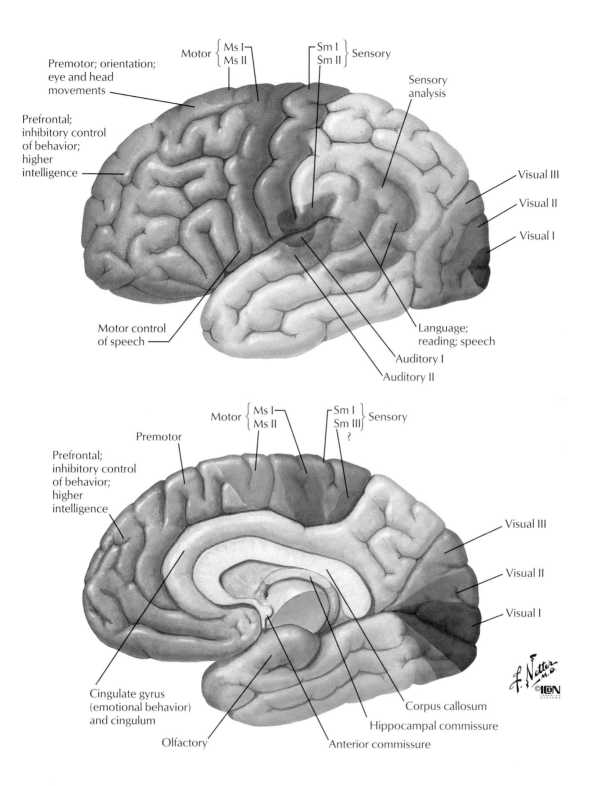

FIGURE 2.19 CEREBRAL CORTEX: LOCALIZATION OF FUNCTION AND ASSOCIATION PATHWAYS

The cerebral cortex is organized into functional regions. In addition to specific areas devoted to sensory and motor functions, there are areas that integrate information from multiple sources. The cerebral cortex participates in advanced intellectual functions, including aspects of memory storage and recall, language, higher cognitive functions, conscious perception, sensory integration, and planning/execution of complex motor activity. General cortical areas associated with these functions are illustrated.

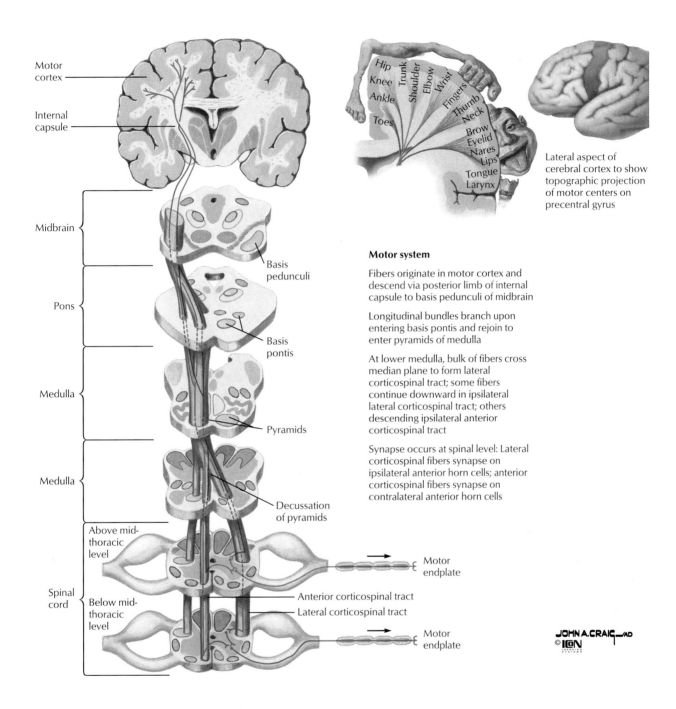

Motor cortex

Internal capsule

Midbrain

Pons

Medulla

Medulla

Above mid-thoracic level

Spinal cord

Below mid-thoracic level

Basis pedunculi

Basis pontis

Pyramids

Decussation of pyramids

Motor endplate

Anterior corticospinal tract
Lateral corticospinal tract

Motor endplate

Hip
Knee
Trunk
Shoulder
Elbow
Wrist
Ankle
Fingers
Toes
Thumb
Neck
Brow
Eyelid
Nares
Lips
Tongue
Larynx

Lateral aspect of cerebral cortex to show topographic projection of motor centers on precentral gyrus

Motor system

Fibers originate in motor cortex and descend via posterior limb of internal capsule to basis pedunculi of midbrain

Longitudinal bundles branch upon entering basis pontis and rejoin to enter pyramids of medulla

At lower medulla, bulk of fibers cross median plane to form lateral corticospinal tract; some fibers continue downward in ipsilateral lateral corticospinal tract; others descending ipsilateral anterior corticospinal tract

Synapse occurs at spinal level: Lateral corticospinal fibers synapse on ipsilateral anterior horn cells; anterior corticospinal fibers synapse on contralateral anterior horn cells

JOHN A. CRAIG—AD
©ICON LEARNING SYSTEMS

FIGURE 2.20   CORTICOSPINAL TRACTS

The corticospinal, or pyramidal, tract is the major motor tract that controls voluntary movement of the skeletal muscles, especially skilled movements of distal muscles of the limbs. All structures from the cerebral cortex to the anterior horn cells in the spinal cord constitute the upper portion of the system (upper motor neuron). The anterior horn cells and their associated axons constitute the lower portion of the system (lower motor neuron).

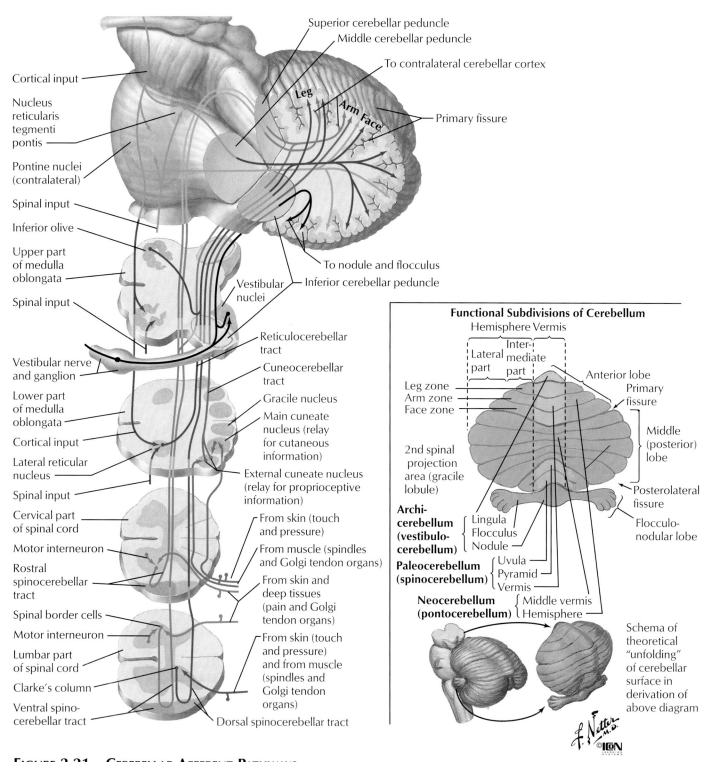

FIGURE 2.21   CEREBELLAR AFFERENT PATHWAYS

The cerebellum plays an important role in coordinating movement. It receives sensory information and then influences descending motor pathways to produce fine, smooth, and coordinated motion. The cerebellum is divided into three general areas: archicerebellum (also called vestibulocerebellum) paleocerebellum (also called spinocerebellum) and the neocerebellum (also called the cerebrocerebellum). The archicerebellum is primarily involved in controlling posture and balance, as well as the movement of the head and eyes. It receives afferent signals from the vestibular apparatus and then sends efferent fibers to the appropriate descending motor pathways. The paleocere-

bellum primarily controls movement of the proximal portions of the limbs. It receives sensory information on limb position and muscle tone and then modifies and coordinates these movements through efferent pathways to the appropriate descending motor pathways. The neocerebellum is the largest portion of the cerebellum, and it coordinates the movement of the distal portions of the limbs. It receives input from the cerebral cortex and thus helps in the planning of motor activity (e.g., seeing a pencil and then planning and executing the movement of the arm and hand to pick it up).

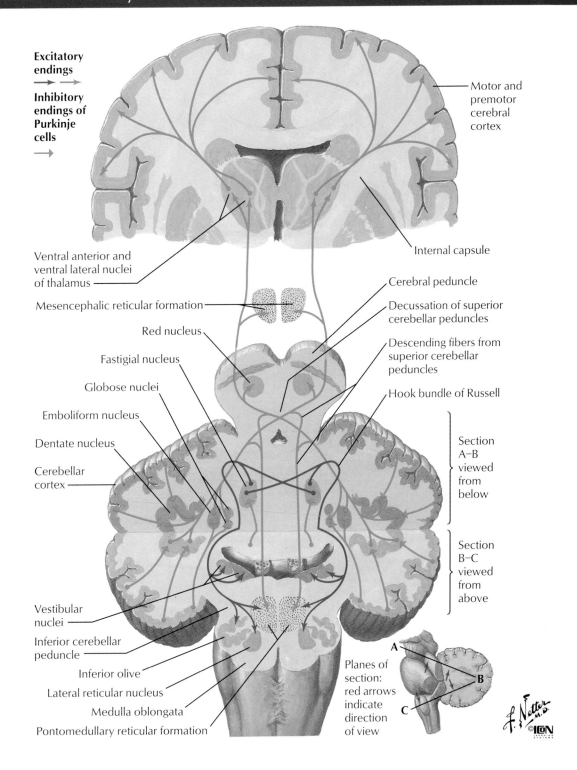

Excitatory
endings
→ →

Inhibitory
endings of
Purkinje
cells
→

Motor and
premotor
cerebral
cortex

Internal capsule

Ventral anterior and
ventral lateral nuclei
of thalamus

Mesencephalic reticular formation

Red nucleus

Fastigial nucleus

Globose nuclei

Emboliform nucleus

Dentate nucleus

Cerebellar
cortex

Cerebral peduncle

Decussation of superior
cerebellar peduncles

Descending fibers from
superior cerebellar
peduncles

Hook bundle of Russell

Section
A–B
viewed
from
below

Section
B–C
viewed
from
above

Vestibular
nuclei

Inferior cerebellar
peduncle

Inferior olive

Lateral reticular nucleus

Medulla oblongata

Pontomedullary reticular formation

Planes of
section:
red arrows
indicate
direction
of view

A

B

C

FIGURE 2.22   CEREBELLAR EFFERENT PATHWAYS

The cerebellum plays an important role in coordinating movement. It influences descending motor pathways to produce fine, smooth, and coordinated motion. The archicerebellum is primarily involved in controlling posture and balance and movement of the head and eyes. It sends efferent fibers to the appropriate descending motor pathways. The paleocerebellum primarily controls movement of the proximal portions of the limbs. It modifies and coordinates these movements through efferent pathways to the appropriate descending motor pathways. The neocerebellum coordinates the movement of the distal portions of the limbs. It helps in the planning of motor activity (e.g., seeing a pencil and then planning and executing the movement of the arm and hand to pick it up).

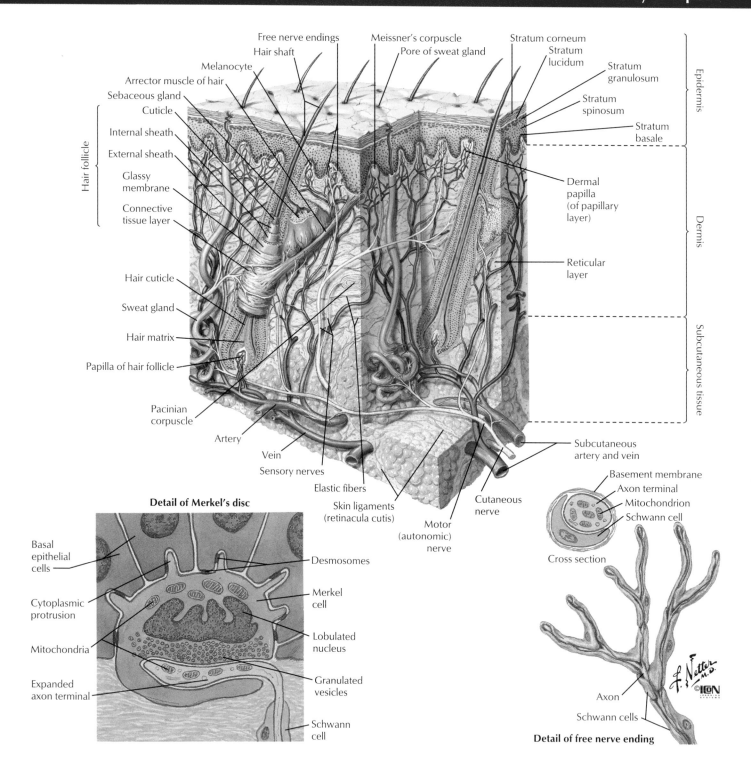

Detail of Merkel's disc

Cross section

Detail of free nerve ending

FIGURE 2.23   SKIN AND CUTANEOUS RECEPTORS

Cutaneous receptors respond to touch (mechanoreceptors), pain (nociceptors), and temperature (thermoreceptors). Several different types of receptors are present in skin. Meissner's corpuscles have small receptive fields and respond best to stimuli that are applied at low frequency (i.e., flutter). The pacinian corpuscles are located in the subcutaneous tissue and have large receptive fields. They respond best to high-frequency stimulation (i.e., vibration). Merkel's discs have small receptive fields and respond to touch and pressure (i.e., indenting the skin). Ruffini's corpuscles have large receptive fields, and they also respond to touch and pressure. Free nerve endings respond to pain and temperature.

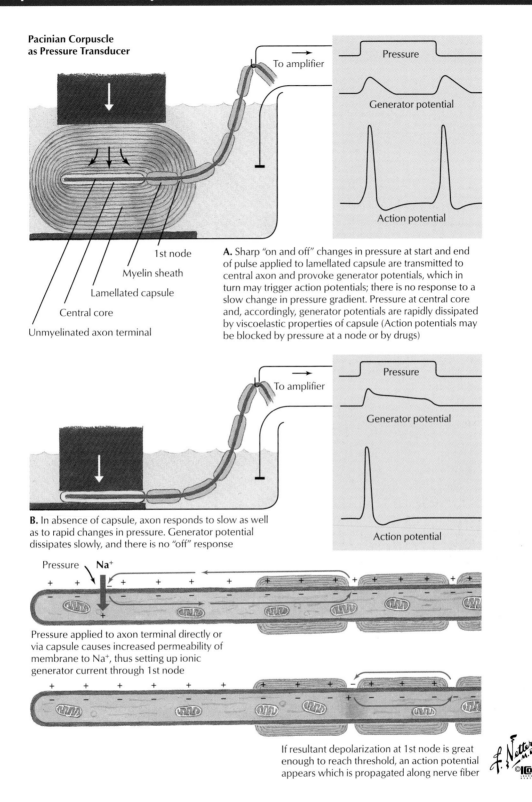

**Pacinian Corpuscle
as Pressure Transducer**

To amplifier

Pressure

Generator potential

Action potential

1st node

Myelin sheath

Lamellated capsule

Central core

Unmyelinated axon terminal

A. Sharp "on and off" changes in pressure at start and end of pulse applied to lamellated capsule are transmitted to central axon and provoke generator potentials, which in turn may trigger action potentials; there is no response to a slow change in pressure gradient. Pressure at central core and, accordingly, generator potentials are rapidly dissipated by viscoelastic properties of capsule (Action potentials may be blocked by pressure at a node or by drugs)

To amplifier

Pressure

Generator potential

Action potential

B. In absence of capsule, axon responds to slow as well as to rapid changes in pressure. Generator potential dissipates slowly, and there is no "off" response

Pressure   **Na⁺**

Pressure applied to axon terminal directly or via capsule causes increased permeability of membrane to Na⁺, thus setting up ionic generator current through 1st node

If resultant depolarization at 1st node is great enough to reach threshold, an action potential appears which is propagated along nerve fiber

FIGURE 2.24   PACINIAN CORPUSCLE

Pacinian corpuscles are mechanoreceptors that transduce mechanical forces (displacement, pressure, vibration) into action potentials that are conveyed centrally by afferent nerve fibers. As the viscoelastic lamellae are displaced, the unmyelinated axon terminal membrane's ionic permeability is increased until it is capable of producing a "generator potential." As demonstrated in the figure, pacinian corpuscles respond to the beginning and end of a mechanical force while the concentric lamellae dissipate slow changes in pressure. In the absence of the capsule, the generator potential decays slowly and yields only a single action potential.

Spinal Effector Mechanisms

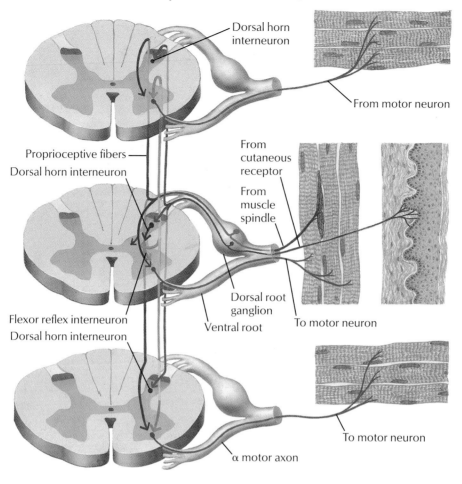

Dorsal horn interneuron

From motor neuron

Proprioceptive fibers

Dorsal horn interneuron

From cutaneous receptor

From muscle spindle

Dorsal root ganglion

To motor neuron

Flexor reflex interneuron

Dorsal horn interneuron

Ventral root

α motor axon

To motor neuron

Schematic representation of motor neurons

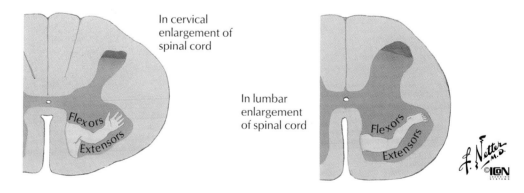

In cervical enlargement of spinal cord

Flexors

Extensors

In lumbar enlargement of spinal cord

Flexors

Extensors

FIGURE 2.25   PROPRIOCEPTION: SPINAL EFFECTOR MECHANISM

Position sense or proprioception involves input from cutaneous mechanoreceptors, Golgi tendon organs, and muscle spindles (middle figure of upper panel). Both monosynaptic reflex pathways (middle figure of upper panel) and polysynaptic pathways involving several spinal cord segments (top and bottom figures of upper panel) initiate muscle contraction reflexes. The lower panel shows the somatotopic distribution of the motor neuron cell bodies in the ventral horn of the spinal cord that innervate limb muscles (flexor and extensor muscles of upper and lower limbs).

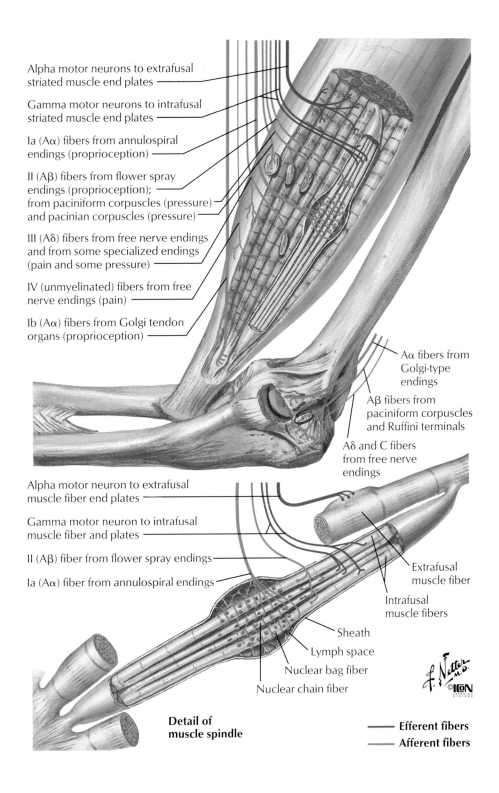

Alpha motor neurons to extrafusal striated muscle end plates

Gamma motor neurons to intrafusal striated muscle end plates

Ia (Aα) fibers from annulospiral endings (proprioception)

II (Aβ) fibers from flower spray endings (proprioception); from paciniform corpuscles (pressure) and pacinian corpuscles (pressure)

III (Aδ) fibers from free nerve endings and from some specialized endings (pain and some pressure)

IV (unmyelinated) fibers from free nerve endings (pain)

Ib (Aα) fibers from Golgi tendon organs (proprioception)

Aα fibers from Golgi-type endings

Aβ fibers from paciniform corpuscles and Ruffini terminals

Aδ and C fibers from free nerve endings

Alpha motor neuron to extrafusal muscle fiber end plates

Gamma motor neuron to intrafusal muscle fiber and plates

II (Aβ) fiber from flower spray endings

Ia (Aα) fiber from annulospiral endings

Extrafusal muscle fiber

Intrafusal muscle fibers

Sheath

Lymph space

Nuclear bag fiber

Nuclear chain fiber

Detail of muscle spindle

—— Efferent fibers
—— Afferent fibers

FIGURE 2.26   MUSCLE AND JOINT RECEPTORS

Muscle spindles and Golgi tendon organs send afferent signals to the brain to convey the position of limbs and help coordinate muscle movement. Muscle spindles convey information on muscle tension and contraction (dynamic forces) and muscle length (static forces). The nuclear bag fibers respond to both dynamic and static forces, whereas the nuclear chain fibers respond to static forces. Intrafusal fibers maintain appropriate tension on the nuclear bag and nuclear chain fibers. If the muscle tension is too great (e.g., overstretching of muscle or too heavy a load), activation of the Golgi tendon organ causes a reflex relaxation of the muscle.

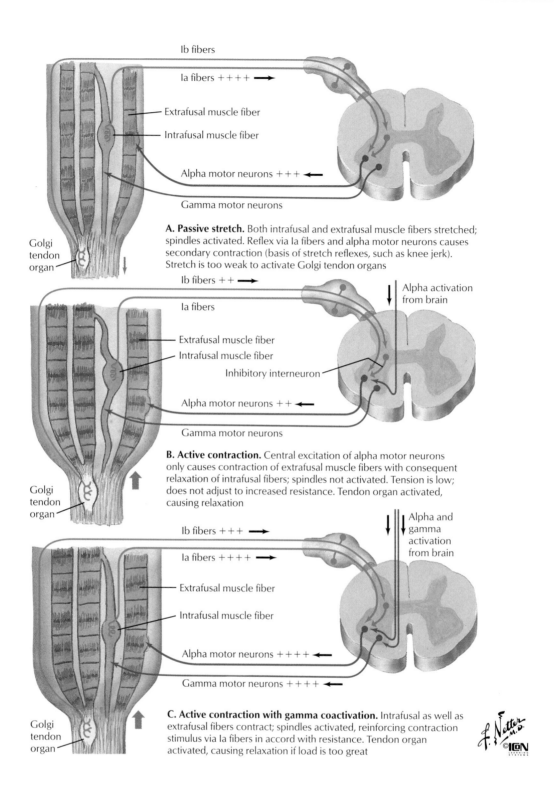

Ib fibers

Ia fibers ++++ →

Extrafusal muscle fiber

Intrafusal muscle fiber

Alpha motor neurons +++ ←

Gamma motor neurons

Golgi tendon organ

A. Passive stretch. Both intrafusal and extrafusal muscle fibers stretched; spindles activated. Reflex via Ia fibers and alpha motor neurons causes secondary contraction (basis of stretch reflexes, such as knee jerk). Stretch is too weak to activate Golgi tendon organs

Ib fibers ++ →

Ia fibers

Alpha activation from brain

Extrafusal muscle fiber

Intrafusal muscle fiber

Inhibitory interneuron

Alpha motor neurons ++ ←

Gamma motor neurons

Golgi tendon organ

B. Active contraction. Central excitation of alpha motor neurons only causes contraction of extrafusal muscle fibers with consequent relaxation of intrafusal fibers; spindles not activated. Tension is low; does not adjust to increased resistance. Tendon organ activated, causing relaxation

Ib fibers +++ →

Ia fibers ++++ →

Alpha and gamma activation from brain

Extrafusal muscle fiber

Intrafusal muscle fiber

Alpha motor neurons ++++ ←

Gamma motor neurons ++++ ←

Golgi tendon organ

C. Active contraction with gamma coactivation. Intrafusal as well as extrafusal fibers contract; spindles activated, reinforcing contraction stimulus via Ia fibers in accord with resistance. Tendon organ activated, causing relaxation if load is too great

FIGURE 2.27 PROPRIOCEPTIVE REFLEX CONTROL OF MUSCLE TENSION

Interaction of the muscle spindle and Golgi tendon organ during passive stretch of a muscle (panel A) and during a contraction (panels B and C).

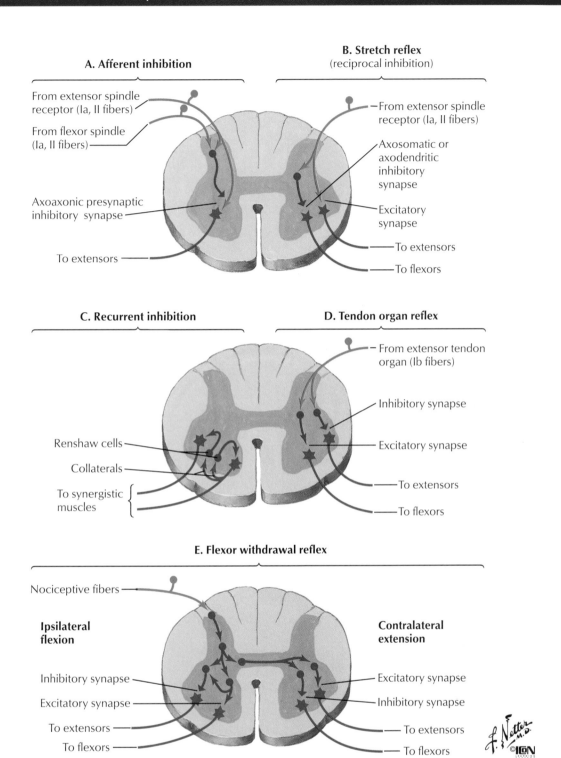

A. Afferent inhibition

From extensor spindle receptor (Ia, II fibers)

From flexor spindle (Ia, II fibers)

Axoaxonic presynaptic inhibitory synapse

To extensors

B. Stretch reflex (reciprocal inhibition)

From extensor spindle receptor (Ia, II fibers)

Axosomatic or axodendritic inhibitory synapse

Excitatory synapse

To extensors

To flexors

C. Recurrent inhibition

Renshaw cells

Collaterals

To synergistic muscles

D. Tendon organ reflex

From extensor tendon organ (Ib fibers)

Inhibitory synapse

Excitatory synapse

To extensors

To flexors

E. Flexor withdrawal reflex

Nociceptive fibers

Ipsilateral flexion

Inhibitory synapse

Excitatory synapse

To extensors

To flexors

Contralateral extension

Excitatory synapse

Inhibitory synapse

To extensors

To flexors

FIGURE 2.28   SPINAL REFLEX PATHWAYS

Summary of the spinal reflex pathways.

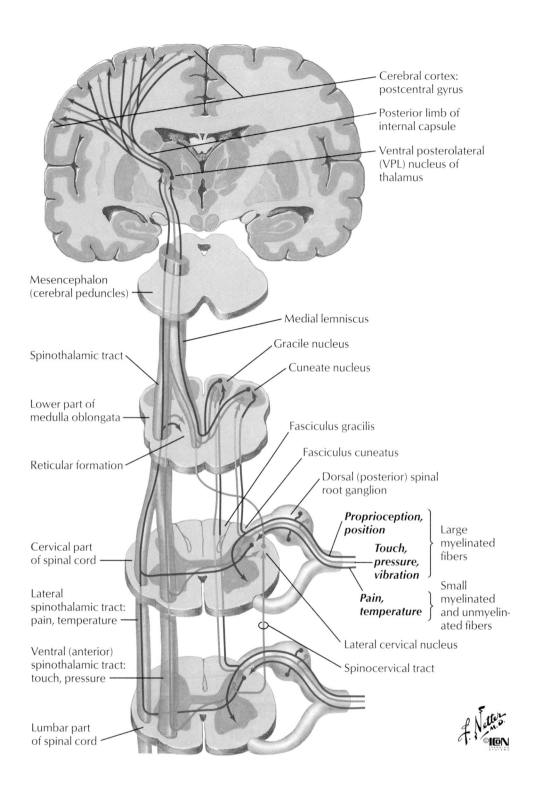

FIGURE 2.29 SOMESTHETIC SYSTEM OF THE BODY

Pain, temperature, and pressure sensations below the head ultimately are conveyed to the primary somatosensory cortex (postcentral gyrus) by the anterolateral system (spinothalamic and spinoreticular tracts). The fasciculus gracilis and cuneatus of the spinal lemniscal system convey proprioceptive, vibratory, and tactile sensations to the thalamus (ventral posterolateral nucleus), whereas the lateral cervical system mediates some touch, vibratory, and proprioceptive sensations (blue and purple lines show these dual pathways). Ultimately, these fibers ascend as parallel pathways to the thalamus, synapse, and ascend to the cortex.

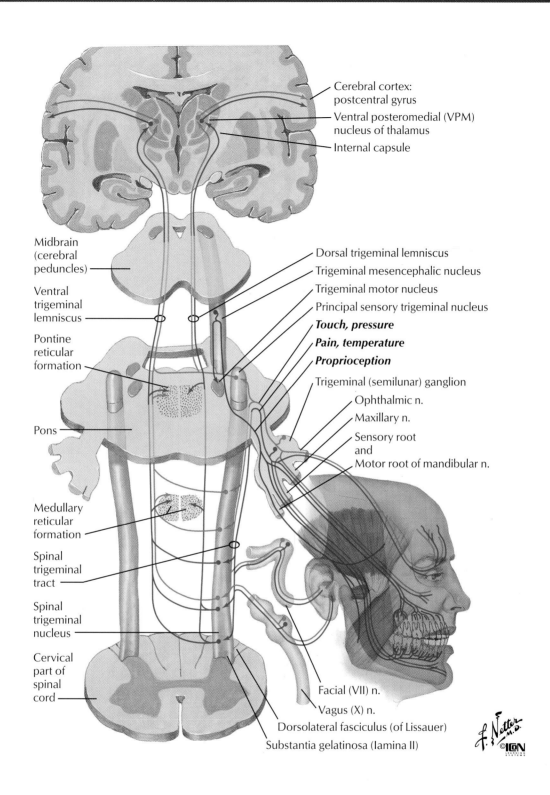

FIGURE 2.30   SOMESTHETIC SYSTEM OF THE HEAD

Nerve cells bodies for touch, pressure, pain, and temperature in the head are in the trigeminal (semilunar) ganglion of the trigeminal (CN V) nerve (blue and red lines in figure). Neuronal cell bodies mediating proprioception reside in the mesencephalic nucleus of CN V (purple fibers). Most relay neurons project to the contralateral VPM nucleus of the thalamus and thence to the postcentral gyrus of the cerebral cortex, where they are somatotopically represented.

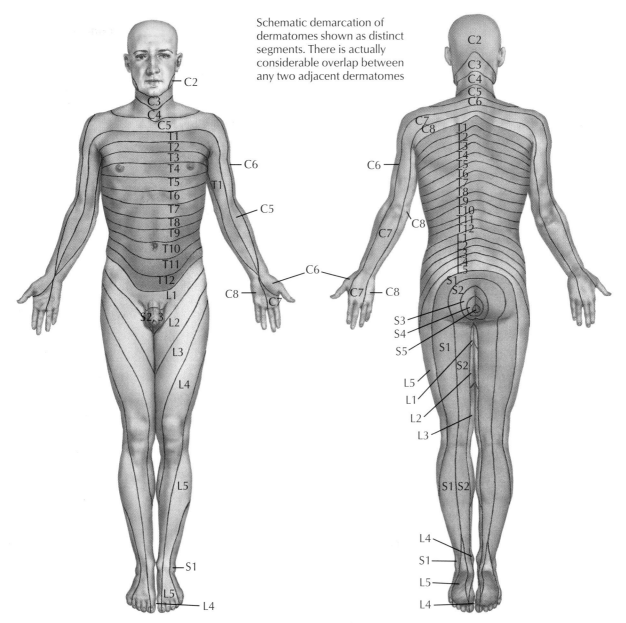

Schematic demarcation of dermatomes shown as distinct segments. There is actually considerable overlap between any two adjacent dermatomes

Levels of principal dermatomes

C5	Clavicles
C5, 6, 7	Lateral parts of upper limbs
C8, T1	Medial sides of upper limbs
C6	Thumb
C6, 7, 8	Hand
C8	Ring and little fingers
T4	Level of nipples

T10	Level of umbilicus
T12	Inguinal or groin regions
L1, 2, 3, 4	Anterior and inner surfaces of lower limbs
L4, 5, S1	Foot
L4	Medial side of great toe
S1, 2, L5	Posterior and outer surfaces of lower limbs
S1	Lateral margin of foot and little toe
S2, 3, 4	Perineum

FIGURE 2.31 DERMATOMES

Sensory information below the head is localized to specific areas of the body, which reflect the distribution of peripheral sensory fibers that convey sensations to the spinal cord through the dorsal roots (sensory nerve cell bodies reside in the corresponding dorsal root ganglion). The area of skin subserved by afferent fibers of one dorsal root is called a dermatome. This figure shows the dermatome segments and lists key dermatome levels used by clinicians. Variability and overlap occur, so all dermatome segments are only approximations.

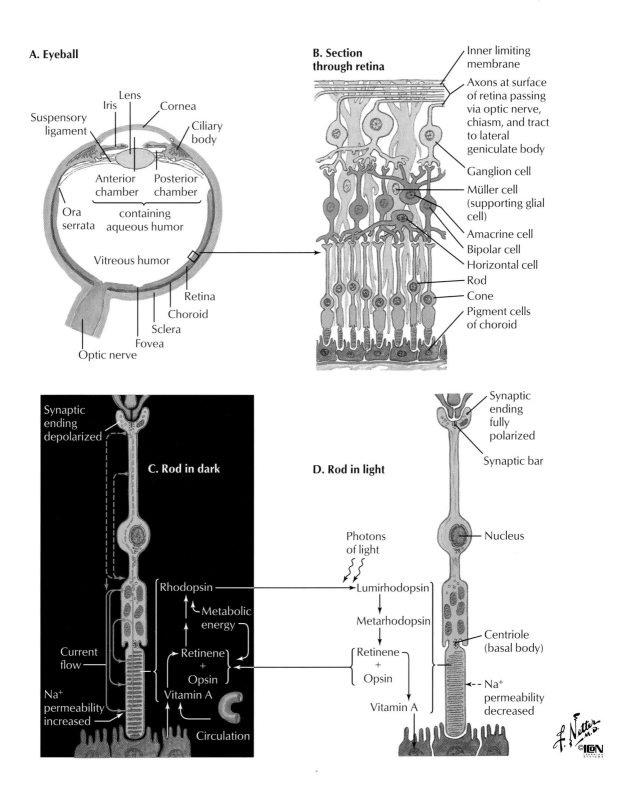

A. Eyeball

Suspensory ligament
Iris
Lens
Cornea
Ciliary body
Anterior chamber
Posterior chamber
Ora serrata
containing aqueous humor
Vitreous humor
Retina
Choroid
Sclera
Fovea
Optic nerve

B. Section through retina

Inner limiting membrane
Axons at surface of retina passing via optic nerve, chiasm, and tract to lateral geniculate body
Ganglion cell
Müller cell (supporting glial cell)
Amacrine cell
Bipolar cell
Horizontal cell
Rod
Cone
Pigment cells of choroid

C. Rod in dark

Synaptic ending depolarized
Current flow
Na⁺ permeability increased
Rhodopsin
Metabolic energy
Retinene + Opsin
Vitamin A
Circulation

D. Rod in light

Synaptic ending fully polarized
Synaptic bar
Photons of light
Lumirhodopsin
Metarhodopsin
Retinene + Opsin
Vitamin A
Nucleus
Centriole (basal body)
Na⁺ permeability decreased

FIGURE 2.32   VISUAL RECEPTORS

The rods and cones of the retina transduce light into electrical signals. As illustrated for the rod, light is absorbed by rhodopsin, and through the second messenger cGMP (not shown), Na⁺ channels in the membrane close and the cell hyperpolarizes. Thus, in the dark the cell is depolarized, but it is hyperpolarized in the light. This electrical response to light is distinct from other receptor responses, in which the response to a stimulus results in a depolarization of the receptor cell membrane.

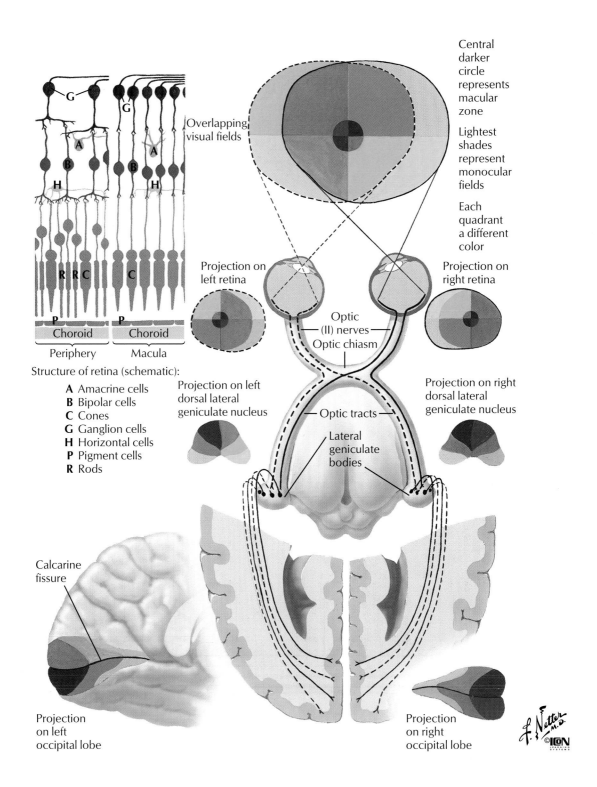

Central darker circle represents macular zone

Lightest shades represent monocular fields

Each quadrant a different color

Overlapping visual fields

Projection on left retina

Projection on right retina

Optic (II) nerves

Optic chiasm

Projection on left dorsal lateral geniculate nucleus

Projection on right dorsal lateral geniculate nucleus

Optic tracts

Lateral geniculate bodies

Calcarine fissure

Projection on left occipital lobe

Projection on right occipital lobe

G
A
B
H
R R C
C
P
Choroid
Choroid
Periphery
Macula

Structure of retina (schematic):

A Amacrine cells
B Bipolar cells
C Cones
G Ganglion cells
H Horizontal cells
P Pigment cells
R Rods

FIGURE 2.33 RETINOGENICULOSTRIATE VISUAL PATHWAY

The retina has two types of photoreceptors: cones that mediate color vision and rods that mediate light perception but with low acuity. The greatest acuity is found in the region of the macula of the retina, where only cones are found (upper left panel). Visual signals are conveyed by the ganglion cells whose axons course in the optic nerves. Visual signals from the nasal retina cross in the optic chiasm while information from the temporal retina remains in the ipsilateral optic tract. Fibers synapse in the lateral geniculate nucleus (visual field is topographically represented here and inverted), and signals are conveyed to the visual cortex on the medial surface of the occipital lobe.

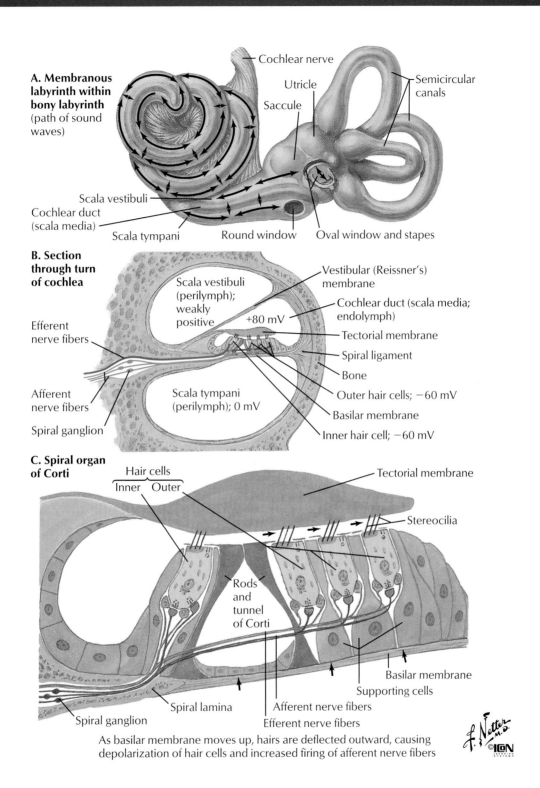

A. Membranous labyrinth within bony labyrinth (path of sound waves)

Cochlear nerve

Utricle

Saccule

Semicircular canals

Scala vestibuli

Cochlear duct (scala media)

Scala tympani

Round window

Oval window and stapes

B. Section through turn of cochlea

Scala vestibuli (perilymph); weakly positive   +80 mV

Vestibular (Reissner's) membrane

Cochlear duct (scala media; endolymph)

Tectorial membrane

Spiral ligament

Bone

Efferent nerve fibers

Afferent nerve fibers

Spiral ganglion

Scala tympani (perilymph); 0 mV

Outer hair cells; −60 mV

Basilar membrane

Inner hair cell; −60 mV

C. Spiral organ of Corti

Hair cells

Inner   Outer

Tectorial membrane

Stereocilia

Rods and tunnel of Corti

Spiral lamina

Spiral ganglion

Afferent nerve fibers

Efferent nerve fibers

Supporting cells

Basilar membrane

As basilar membrane moves up, hairs are deflected outward, causing depolarization of hair cells and increased firing of afferent nerve fibers

---

FIGURE 2.34   COCHLEAR RECEPTORS

The cochlea transduces sound into electrical signals. This is accomplished by the hair cells, which depolarize in response to vibration of the basilar membrane. The basilar membrane moves in response to pressure changes imparted on the oval window of the cochlea in response to vibrations of the tympanic membrane.

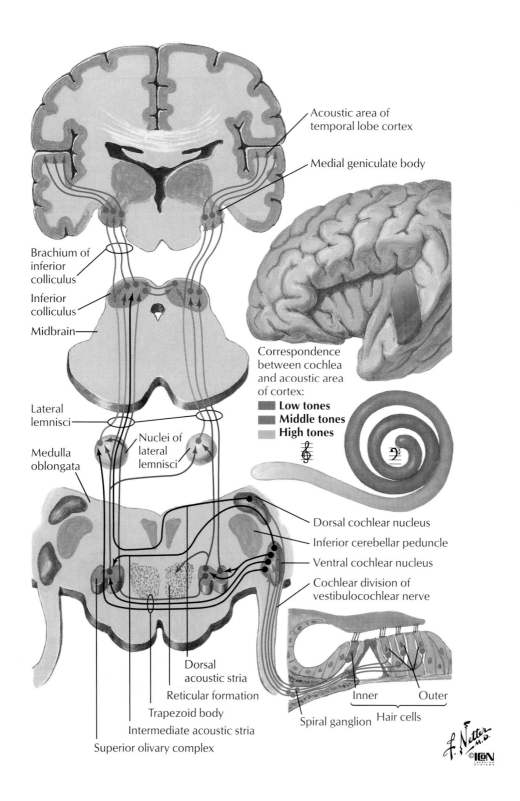

Acoustic area of temporal lobe cortex

Medial geniculate body

Brachium of inferior colliculus

Inferior colliculus

Midbrain

Lateral lemnisci

Nuclei of lateral lemnisci

Medulla oblongata

Correspondence between cochlea and acoustic area of cortex:

Low tones
Middle tones
High tones

Dorsal cochlear nucleus

Inferior cerebellar peduncle

Ventral cochlear nucleus

Cochlear division of vestibulocochlear nerve

Dorsal acoustic stria

Reticular formation

Trapezoid body

Intermediate acoustic stria

Superior olivary complex

Spiral ganglion

Inner   Outer

Hair cells

FIGURE 2.35   AUDITORY PATHWAYS

The cochlea transduces sound into electrical signals. Axons convey these signals to the dorsal and ventral cochlear nuclei, where it is tonotopically organized. Following a series of integrated relay pathways, the ascending pathway projects to the thalamus (medial geniculate bodies) and then the acoustic cortex in the transverse gyrus of the temporal lobe, where information is tonotopically represented (low, middle, and high tones).

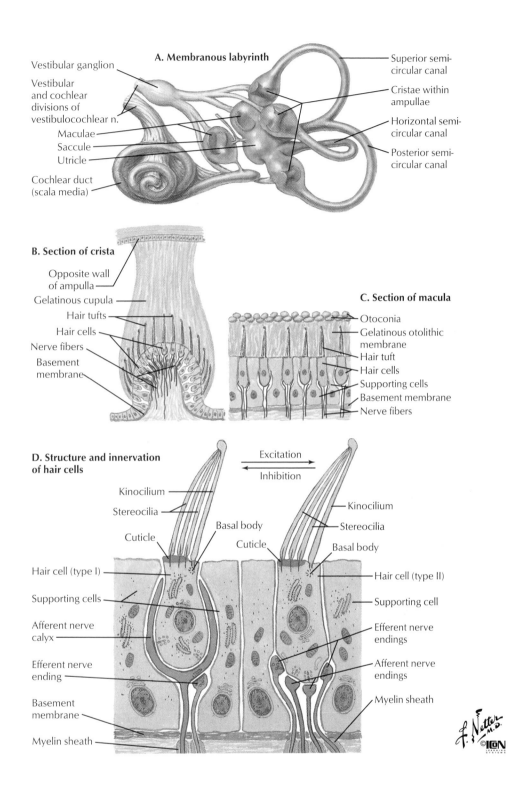

A. Membranous labyrinth

Vestibular ganglion

Vestibular and cochlear divisions of vestibulocochlear n.

Maculae

Saccule

Utricle

Cochlear duct (scala media)

Superior semi-circular canal

Cristae within ampullae

Horizontal semi-circular canal

Posterior semi-circular canal

B. Section of crista

Opposite wall of ampulla

Gelatinous cupula

Hair tufts

Hair cells

Nerve fibers

Basement membrane

C. Section of macula

Otoconia

Gelatinous otolithic membrane

Hair tuft

Hair cells

Supporting cells

Basement membrane

Nerve fibers

D. Structure and innervation of hair cells

Excitation

Inhibition

Kinocilium

Stereocilia

Cuticle

Basal body

Cuticle

Kinocilium

Stereocilia

Basal body

Hair cell (type I)

Supporting cells

Afferent nerve calyx

Efferent nerve ending

Basement membrane

Myelin sheath

Hair cell (type II)

Supporting cell

Efferent nerve endings

Afferent nerve endings

Myelin sheath

FIGURE 2.36 VESTIBULAR RECEPTORS

The vestibular apparatus detects movement of the head in the form of linear and angular acceleration. This information is important for the control of eye movements so that the retina can be provided with a stable visual image. It is also important for the control of posture. The utricle and saccule respond to linear acceleration, such as the pull of gravity. The three semicircular canals are aligned so that the angular movement of the head can be sensed in all planes. The sensory hair cells are located in the maculae of the utricle and saccule and in the cristae within each ampullae.

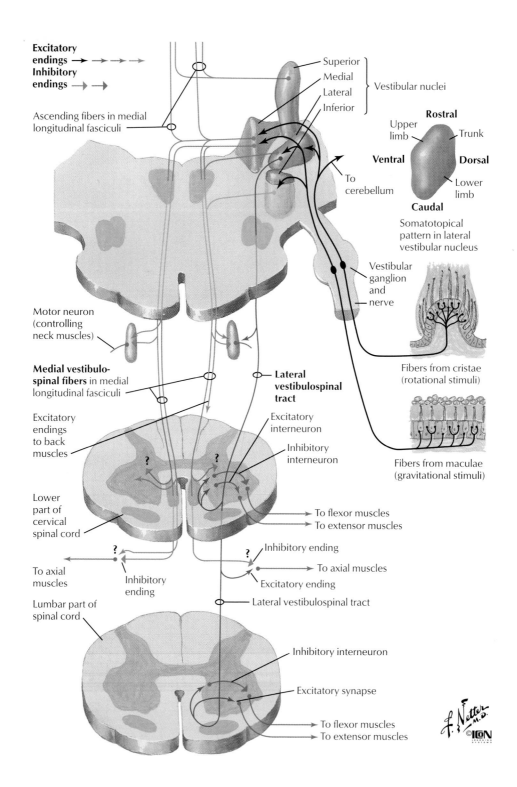

FIGURE 2.37   VESTIBULOSPINAL TRACTS

Sensory input from the vestibular apparatus is used to maintain stability of the head and to maintain balance and posture. Axons convey vestibular information to the vestibular nuclei in the pons, and then secondary axons distribute this information to five sites: spinal cord (muscle control), cerebellum (vermis), reticular formation (vomiting center), extraocular muscles, and cortex (conscious perception). This figure shows only the spinal cord pathways.

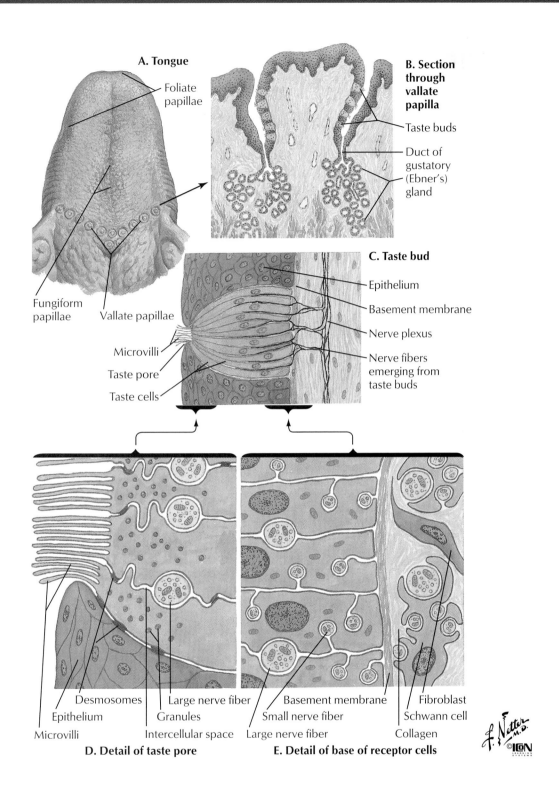

A. Tongue

Foliate papillae

B. Section through vallate papilla

Taste buds

Duct of gustatory (Ebner's) gland

Fungiform papillae

Vallate papillae

C. Taste bud

Epithelium

Basement membrane

Nerve plexus

Nerve fibers emerging from taste buds

Microvilli

Taste pore

Taste cells

Desmosomes

Large nerve fiber

Basement membrane

Fibroblast

Epithelium

Granules

Small nerve fiber

Schwann cell

Microvilli

Intercellular space

Large nerve fiber

Collagen

D. Detail of taste pore

E. Detail of base of receptor cells

FIGURE 2.38 TASTE RECEPTORS

Taste buds on the tongue respond to various chemical stimuli. Taste cells, like neurons, normally have a net negative charge internally and are depolarized by stimuli, thus releasing transmitters that depo-larize neurons connected to the taste cells. A single taste bud can respond to more than one stimulus. The four traditional taste qualities that are sensed are sweet, salty, sour, and bitter.

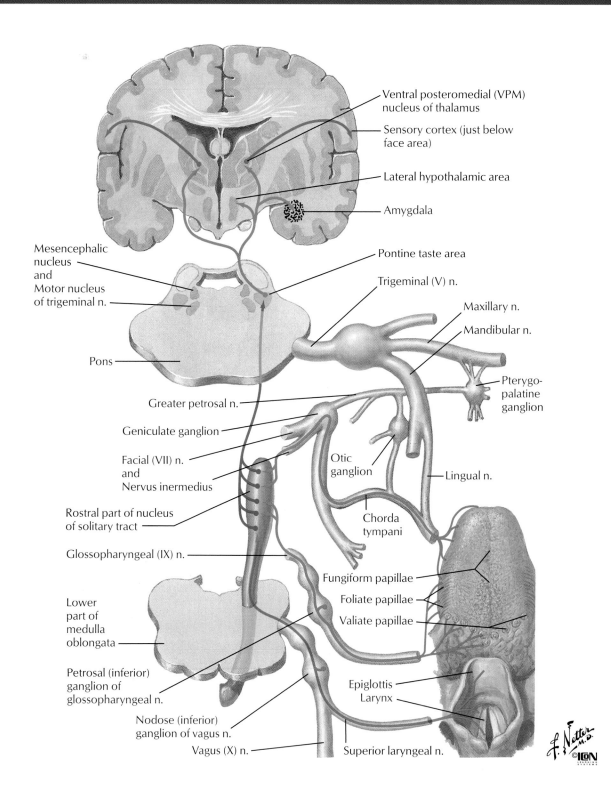

Ventral posteromedial (VPM) nucleus of thalamus

Sensory cortex (just below face area)

Lateral hypothalamic area

Amygdala

Mesencephalic nucleus and Motor nucleus of trigeminal n.

Pontine taste area

Trigeminal (V) n.

Maxillary n.

Mandibular n.

Pons

Pterygo-palatine ganglion

Greater petrosal n.

Geniculate ganglion

Facial (VII) n. and Nervus inermedius

Otic ganglion

Lingual n.

Chorda tympani

Rostral part of nucleus of solitary tract

Glossopharyngeal (IX) n.

Fungiform papillae

Foliate papillae

Valiate papillae

Lower part of medulla oblongata

Petrosal (inferior) ganglion of glossopharyngeal n.

Nodose (inferior) ganglion of vagus n.

Epiglottis

Larynx

Vagus (X) n.

Superior laryngeal n.

FIGURE 2.39 TASTE PATHWAYS

Depicted here are the afferent pathways leading from the taste receptors to the brainstem and, ultimately, to the sensory cortex in the postcentral gyrus.

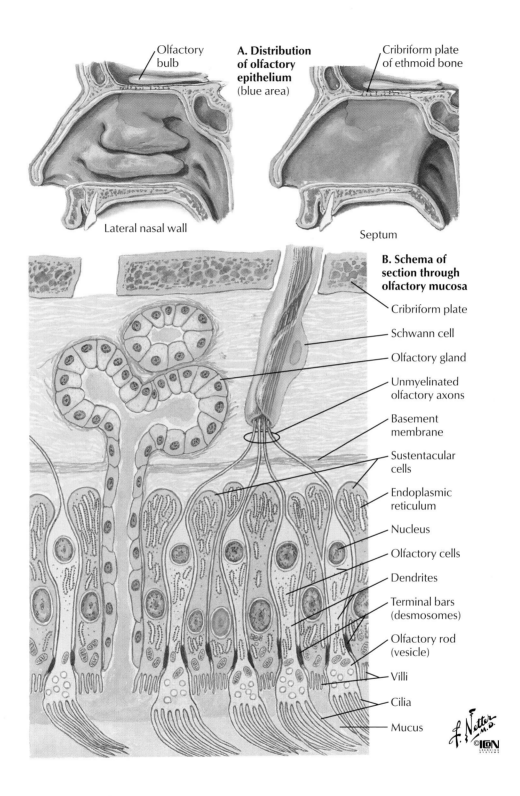

A. Distribution of olfactory epithelium (blue area)

Olfactory bulb

Cribriform plate of ethmoid bone

Lateral nasal wall

Septum

B. Schema of section through olfactory mucosa

- Cribriform plate
- Schwann cell
- Olfactory gland
- Unmyelinated olfactory axons
- Basement membrane
- Sustentacular cells
- Endoplasmic reticulum
- Nucleus
- Olfactory cells
- Dendrites
- Terminal bars (desmosomes)
- Olfactory rod (vesicle)
- Villi
- Cilia
- Mucus

FIGURE 2.40   OLFACTORY RECEPTORS

The sensory cells that make up the olfactory epithelium respond to odorants by depolarizing. Like taste buds, an olfactory cell can respond to more than one odorant. There are six general odor qualities that can be sensed: floral, ethereal (e.g., pears), musky, camphor (e.g., eucalyptus), putrid, and pungent (e.g., vinegar, peppermint).

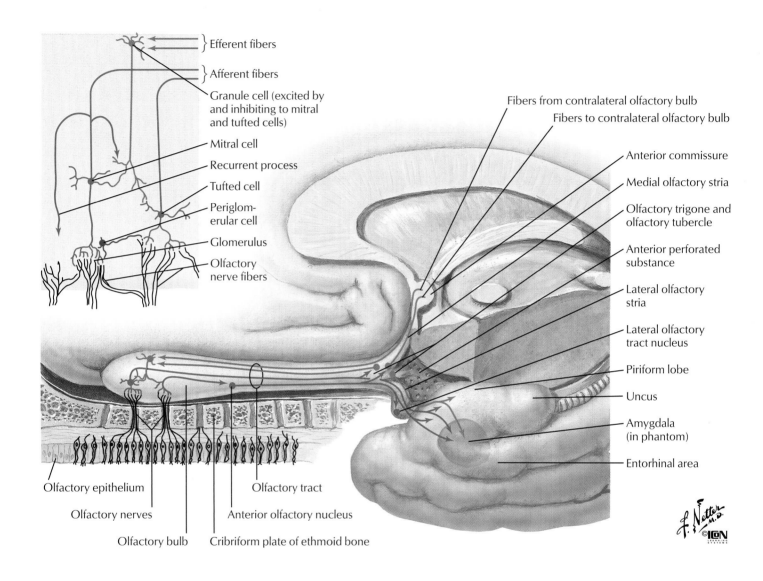

FIGURE 2.41   OLFACTORY PATHWAY

Olfactory stimuli are detected by the nerve fibers of the olfactory epithelium and conveyed to the olfactory bulb (detailed local circuitry shown in upper left panel). Integrated signals pass along the olfactory tract and centrally diverge to pass to the anterior commissure (some efferent projections course to the contralateral olfactory bulb, blue lines) or terminate in the ipsilateral olfactory trigone (olfactory tubercle). Axons then project to the primary olfactory cortex (piriform cortex), entorhinal cortex, and amygdala.

Chapter 3 Muscle Physiology

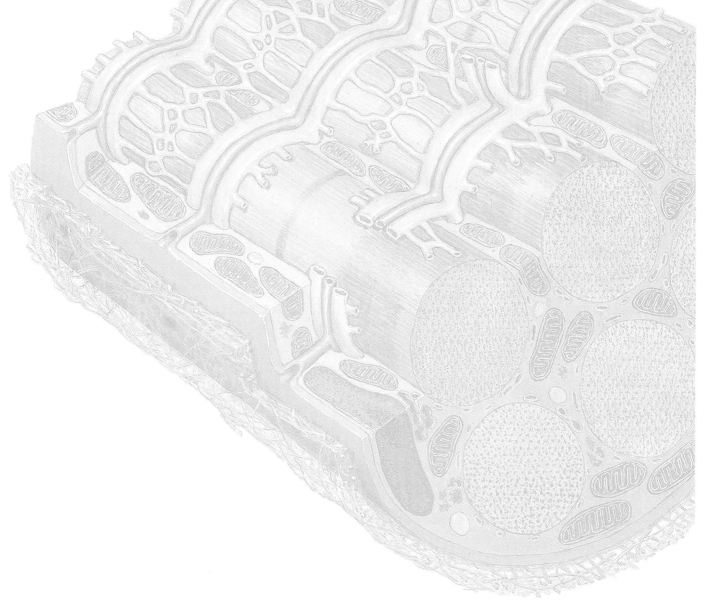

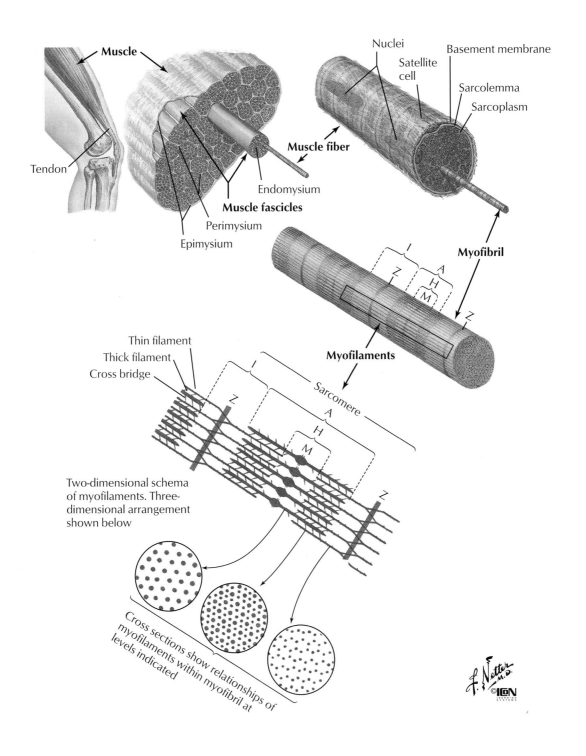

FIGURE 3.1 ORGANIZATION OF SKELETAL MUSCLE

Skeletal muscle is specialized for voluntary movement. The muscle fiber is a multinucleated cell that contains the contractile elements, called myofilaments. The myofilaments are organized as myofibrils within the fiber. Groups of muscle fibers are organized into muscle fascicles, which in turn are grouped to form a muscle. The regular arrangement of the myofibrils gives skeletal muscle a striated appearance under the microscope.

Segment of muscle fiber greatly enlarged to show sarcoplasmic structures and inclusions

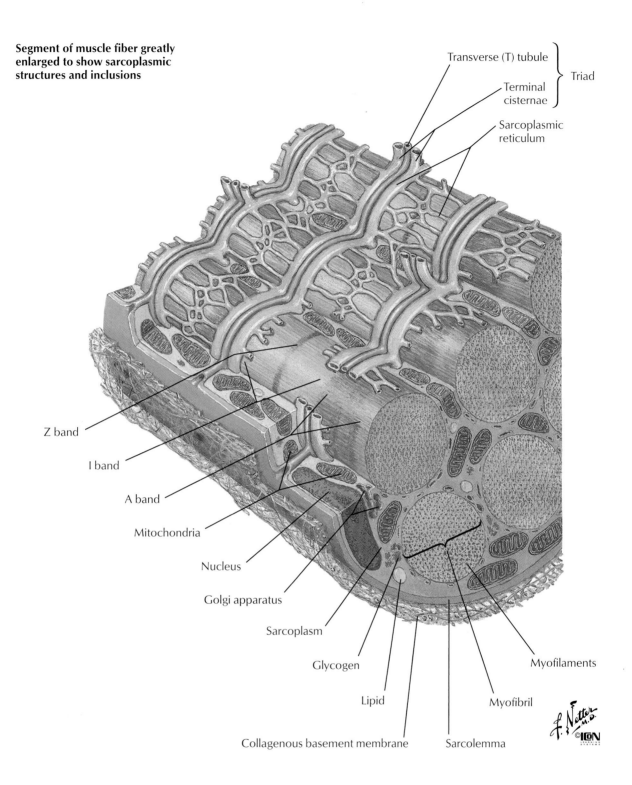

Transverse (T) tubule

Terminal cisternae

Triad

Sarcoplasmic reticulum

Z band

I band

A band

Mitochondria

Nucleus

Golgi apparatus

Sarcoplasm

Glycogen

Lipid

Collagenous basement membrane

Myofilaments

Myofibril

Sarcolemma

FIGURE 3.2 SARCOPLASMIC RETICULUM

The sarcoplasmic reticulum forms an elaborate network within the cell and is the storage site for intracellular Ca^{2+}. The sarcoplasmic reticulum contains Ca^{2+} channels, Ca^{2+}-ATPase, and the low-affinity Ca^{2+}-binding protein calsequestrin.

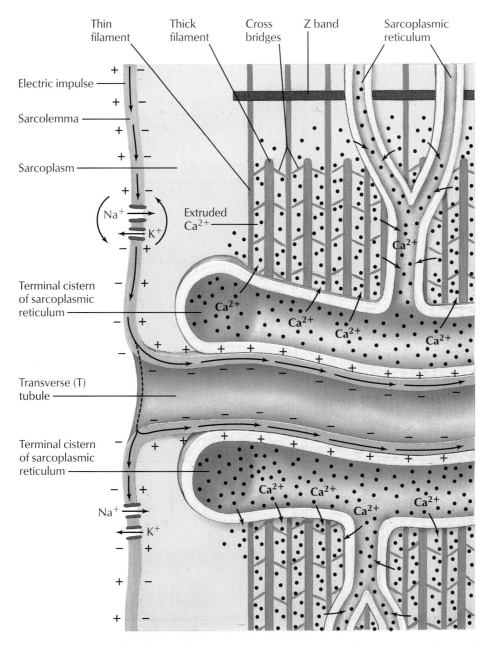

Thin filament · Thick filament · Cross bridges · Z band · Sarcoplasmic reticulum

Electric impulse

Sarcolemma

Sarcoplasm

Na^+ · K^+

Extruded Ca^{2+}

Ca^{2+}

Terminal cistern of sarcoplasmic reticulum

Ca^{2+} · Ca^{2+} · Ca^{2+} · Ca^{2+}

Transverse (T) tubule

Terminal cistern of sarcoplasmic reticulum

Ca^{2+} · Ca^{2+} · Ca^{2+} · Ca^{2+}

Na^+ · K^+

Electric impulse traveling along muscle cell membrane (sarcolemma) from motor endplate (neuromuscular junction) and then along transverse tubules affects sarcoplasmic reticulum, causing extrusion of Ca^{2+} to initiate contraction by "rowing" action of cross bridges, sliding filaments past one another

FIGURE 3.3   EXCITATION-CONTRACTION COUPLING

Impulses from motor neurons release acetylcholine (ACh) at the neuromuscular junction. The ACh receptor on the plasma membrane of the muscle fiber is a cation channel that opens when it binds ACh. As extracellular Na^+ enters the cell through the cation channel, the membrane depolarizes and an action potential is generated. The action potential spreads across the fiber and travels down specialized invaginations called *transverse* (T) *tubules*. The T tubules are in close apposition to the terminal cisternae of the sarcoplasmic reticulum (SR), and the spreading wave of depolarization along the T tubule causes Ca^{2+} release from the SR. Other regions of the SR also contain Ca^{2+}-ATPase, which serves to rapidly reaccumulate the released Ca^{2+} and end the contraction.

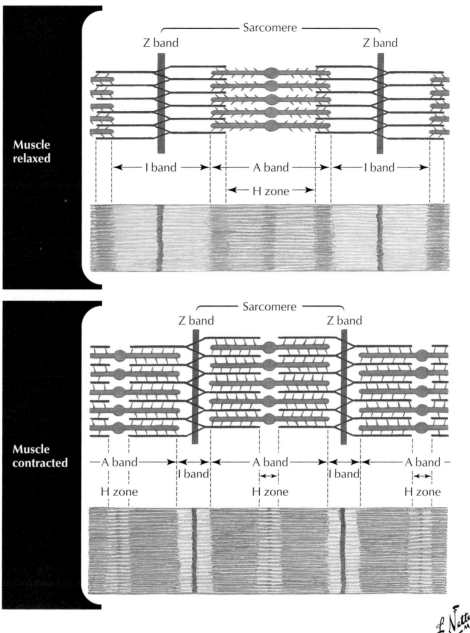

During muscle contraction, thin filaments of each myofibril slide deeply between thick filaments, bringing Z bands closer together and shortening sarcomeres. A bands remain same width, but I bands narrowed. H zones also narrowed or disappear as thin filaments encroach upon them. Myofibrils, and consequently muscle fibers (muscle cells), fascicles, and muscle as whole grow thicker. During relaxation, reverse occurs

FIGURE 3.4   MUSCLE CONTRACTION AND RELAXATION

The sliding of the actin and myosin filaments past one another results in contraction. This sliding action is the result of the cyclical binding (cross-bridge formation) of actin and myosin.

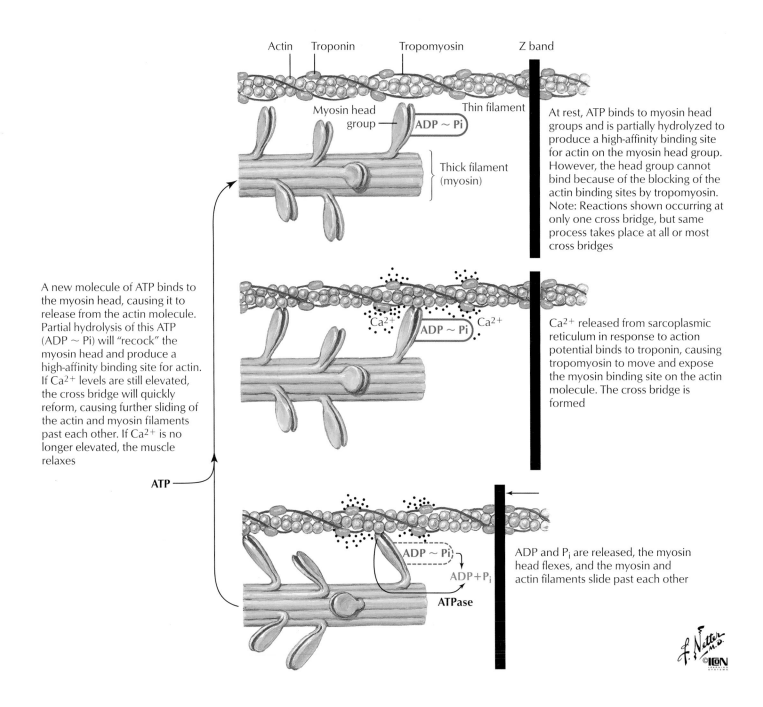

Actin   Troponin   Tropomyosin   Z band

Myosin head group — ADP ~ Pi

Thin filament

Thick filament (myosin)

At rest, ATP binds to myosin head groups and is partially hydrolyzed to produce a high-affinity binding site for actin on the myosin head group. However, the head group cannot bind because of the blocking of the actin binding sites by tropomyosin. Note: Reactions shown occurring at only one cross bridge, but same process takes place at all or most cross bridges

A new molecule of ATP binds to the myosin head, causing it to release from the actin molecule. Partial hydrolysis of this ATP (ADP ~ Pi) will "recock" the myosin head and produce a high-affinity binding site for actin. If Ca^{2+} levels are still elevated, the cross bridge will quickly reform, causing further sliding of the actin and myosin filaments past each other. If Ca^{2+} is no longer elevated, the muscle relaxes

Ca^{2+} ADP ~ Pi Ca^{2+}

Ca^{2+} released from sarcoplasmic reticulum in response to action potential binds to troponin, causing tropomyosin to move and expose the myosin binding site on the actin molecule. The cross bridge is formed

ATP —

ADP ~ Pi

ADP + Pi

ATPase

ADP and P_i are released, the myosin head flexes, and the myosin and actin filaments slide past each other

FIGURE 3.5   BIOCHEMICAL MECHANICS OF MUSCLE CONTRACTION

The contraction of the myofilaments results from the interaction of actin and myosin. In the resting state, myosin is prevented from interacting with actin because the regulatory protein tropomyosin overlies the myosin-binding sites on the actin filament. When Ca^{2+} is released from the SR, it binds to another regulatory protein, tro-ponin. Troponin is closely associated with tropomyosin, and when it binds Ca^{2+}, it undergoes an conformational change that moves the tropomyosin and exposes the myosin-binding sites on the actin filament.

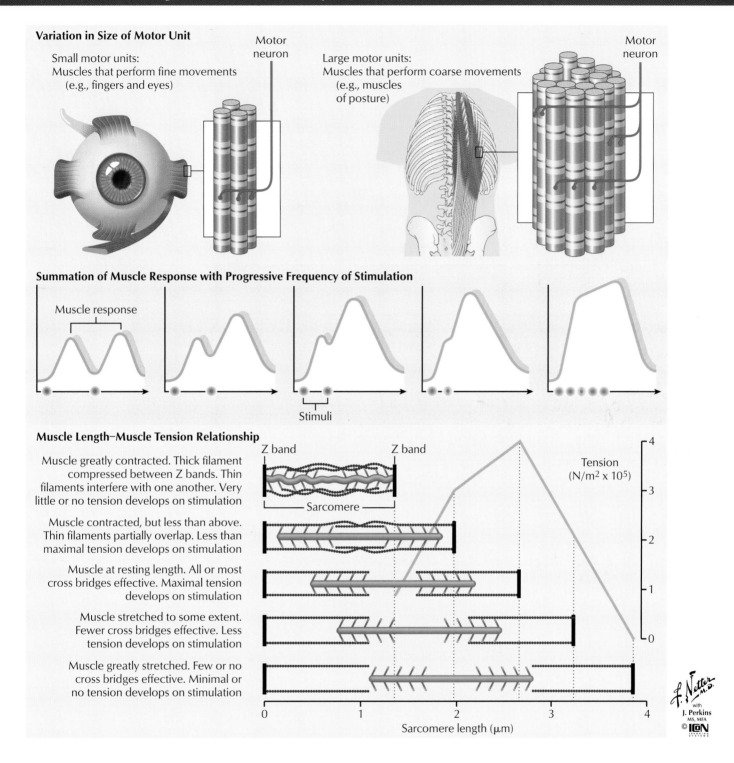

Variation in Size of Motor Unit

Small motor units:
Muscles that perform fine movements
(e.g., fingers and eyes)

Motor neuron

Large motor units:
Muscles that perform coarse movements
(e.g., muscles of posture)

Motor neuron

Summation of Muscle Response with Progressive Frequency of Stimulation

Muscle response

Stimuli

Muscle Length–Muscle Tension Relationship

Muscle greatly contracted. Thick filament compressed between Z bands. Thin filaments interfere with one another. Very little or no tension develops on stimulation

Muscle contracted, but less than above. Thin filaments partially overlap. Less than maximal tension develops on stimulation

Muscle at resting length. All or most cross bridges effective. Maximal tension develops on stimulation

Muscle stretched to some extent. Fewer cross bridges effective. Less tension develops on stimulation

Muscle greatly stretched. Few or no cross bridges effective. Minimal or no tension develops on stimulation

Z band   Z band

Sarcomere

Tension
(N/m^2 x 10^5)

Sarcomere length (μm)

J. Perkins
MS, MFA

FIGURE 3.6   GRADING OF MUSCLE TENSION AND LENGTH-TENSION RELATIONSHIP

The force or tension generated by skeletal muscle can vary by several mechanisms. First, more motor units can be recruited. As shown in the upper panel, a motor unit represents all the muscle fibers innervated by a single motor neuron. The firing of more motor neurons will result in the contraction of a larger number of motor units and thereby generate more tension by the muscle. Second, the frequency of stimulation of a single muscle fiber can increase the tension developed by that fiber. This process, called summation, is shown in the middle panel and results from the sustained elevation of intracellular [Ca^{2+}] that results from high-frequency stimulation. Finally, the tension generated by a single twitch varies as a function of sarcomere length. As shown in the lower panel, the degree of overlap of the thin and thick filaments varies as a function of sarcomere length. This in turn affects the number of cross bridges formed and thus tension developed.

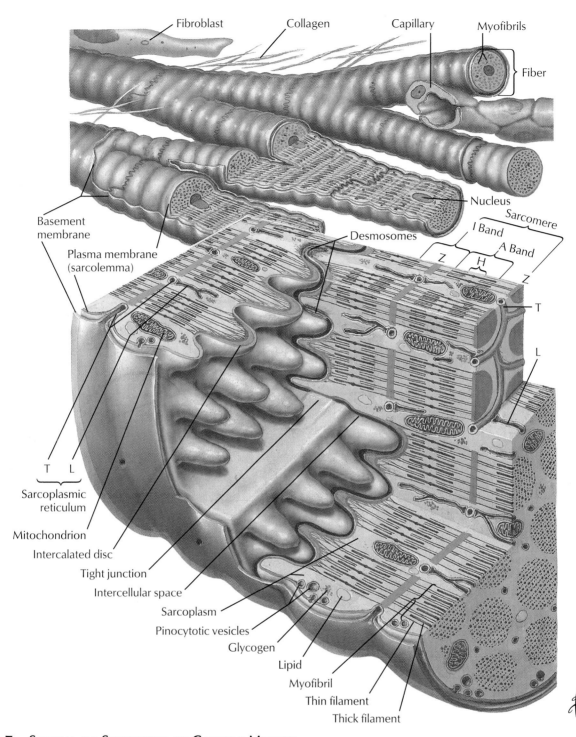

FIGURE 3.7   SCHEMA OF STRUCTURE OF CARDIAC MUSCLE

Cardiac muscle, like skeletal muscle, is striated in appearance, reflecting the presence of the regularly arranged actin and myosin filaments. Cardiac muscle fibers are branched and electrically coupled to one another by gap junctions, which are located in the intercalated discs. The plasma membrane of the cardiac cell (myocyte) contains transverse (T) tubules like skeletal muscle. However, the sarcoplasmic reticulum is not as elaborate as in skeletal muscle, and dyads (rather than triads) are formed between the T tubules and sarcoplasmic reticulum.

Excitation-contraction coupling in cardiac muscle is similar to that of skeletal muscle, as is the process of cross-bridge formation and cycling. Although intracellular Ca^{2+} levels control contraction in both skeletal and cardiac muscle, there are some important differences. Skeletal muscle contraction is dependent on the release of Ca^{2+} from the sarcoplasmic reticulum, and changes in extracellular $[Ca^{2+}]$ do not appreciably alter the strength of the skeletal muscle contraction. In contrast, Ca^{2+} entry into the cardiac myocyte from the extracellular fluid is necessary for the release of Ca^{2+} from the sarcoplasmic reticulum, and removal of extracellular Ca^{2+} will decrease the force of contraction. The rate and force of contraction of cardiac myocytes can be increased by β-adrenergic agonists. β-Adrenergic agonists do not have these effects on skeletal muscle.

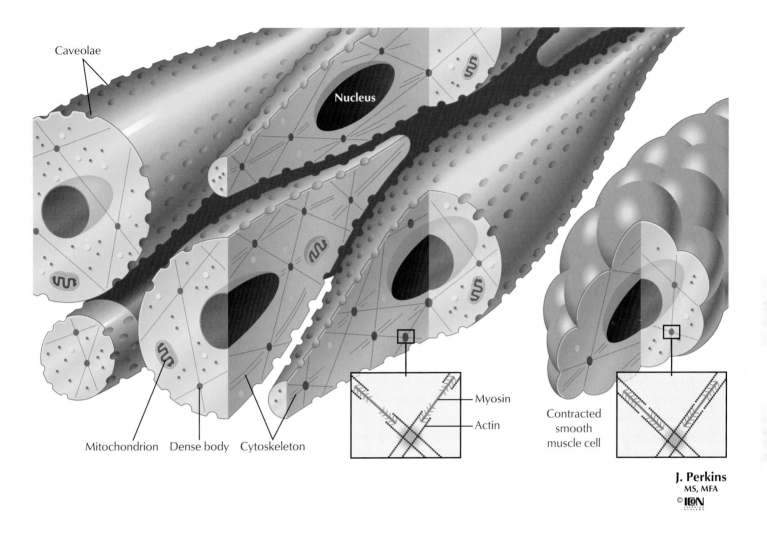

FIGURE 3.8   SMOOTH MUSCLE STRUCTURE

Myofibrils are not found in smooth muscle cells. Instead, actin filaments are anchored to the plasma membrane and to dense bodies within the cytoplasm. Myosin interaction with the actin filaments causes the cell to contract. Smooth muscle cells do not contain T tubules. Instead, caveolae serve a similar function and are a site for entry of extracellular Ca^{2+} into the cell.

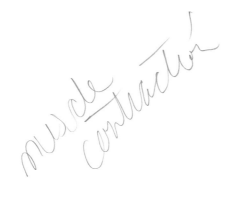

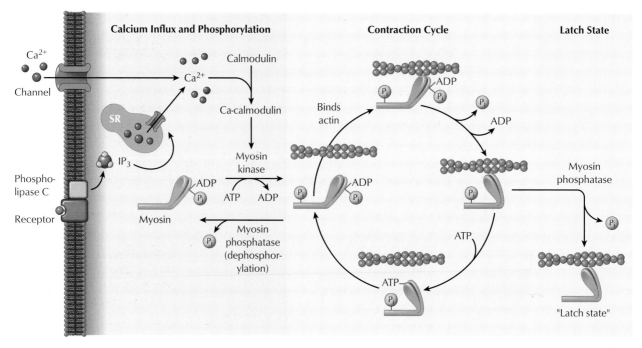

Calcium Influx and Phosphorylation　　　　**Contraction Cycle**　　　　**Latch State**

FIGURE 3.9   EXCITATION-CONTRACTION COUPLING OF SMOOTH MUSCLE

Both extracellular Ca^{2+} and Ca^{2+} release from the sarcoplasmic reticulum regulate smooth muscle contraction. At high intracellular $[Ca^{2+}]$, myosin light-chain kinase (myosin kinase) phosphorylates myosin, which allows actin and myosin to interact. The sliding of actin past myosin in the contraction phase is similar to that of skeletal muscle. As long as the intracellular $[Ca^{2+}]$ is high, the contraction cycle continues. Dephosphorylation of myosin by myosin phosphorylase when it is attached to actin slows the contraction cycle, leading to the latch state (i.e., tonic contraction without hydrolysis of ATP).

CHART 3.1   COMPARISION OF MUSCLE STRUCTURE AND FUNCTION

	Skeletal Muscle	**Cardiac Muscle**	**Smooth Muscle**
Structure			
Morphology	Long; cylindrical	Branched	Spindle or fusiform
Nuclei	Multiple; located peripherally	One (sometimes two); located centrally	One; located centrally
Sarcomere	Yes; striated pattern	Yes; striated pattern	No
T tubules	Yes; forms triad with sarcoplasmic reticulum	Yes; forms dyad with sarcoplasmic reticulum	No; caveolae
Electrical coupling of cells	No	Yes; intercalated discs contain gap junctions	Yes; gap junctions
Regeneration	Yes; via satellite cells	No	Yes
Mitosis	No	No	Yes
Physiology			
Extracellular Ca^{2+} required for contraction	No	Yes	Yes
Regulation of cross-bridge formation	Ca^{2+} binding to troponin	Ca^{2+} binding to troponin	Ca^{2+}-calmodulin activation of myosin kinase and phosphorylation of myosin
Control of contraction	Motor neurons	Autonomic nerves; β-adrenergic agonists	Autonomic nerves; hormones
Summation of twitches by increased stimulus frequency	Yes	No*	Yes
Tension varies with filament overlap	Yes	Yes	Yes

Major differences in structure and function of skeletal, cardiac, and smooth muscle are indicted.
*Cardiac muscle cannot be tetanized, but the force of contraction will increase at high stimulus frequency because of an increase in intracellular $[Ca^{2+}]$, a phenomenon termed "Treppe."

Chapter 4 Cardiovascular Physiology

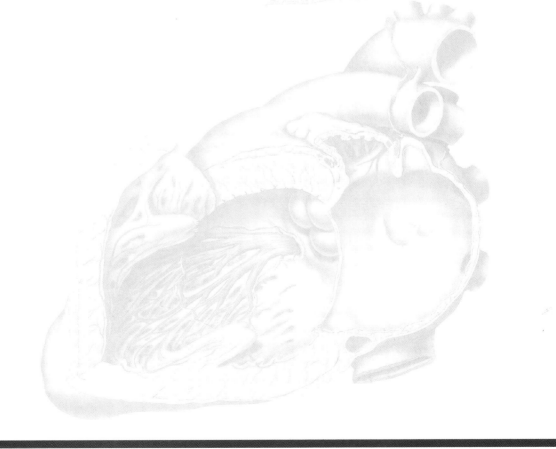

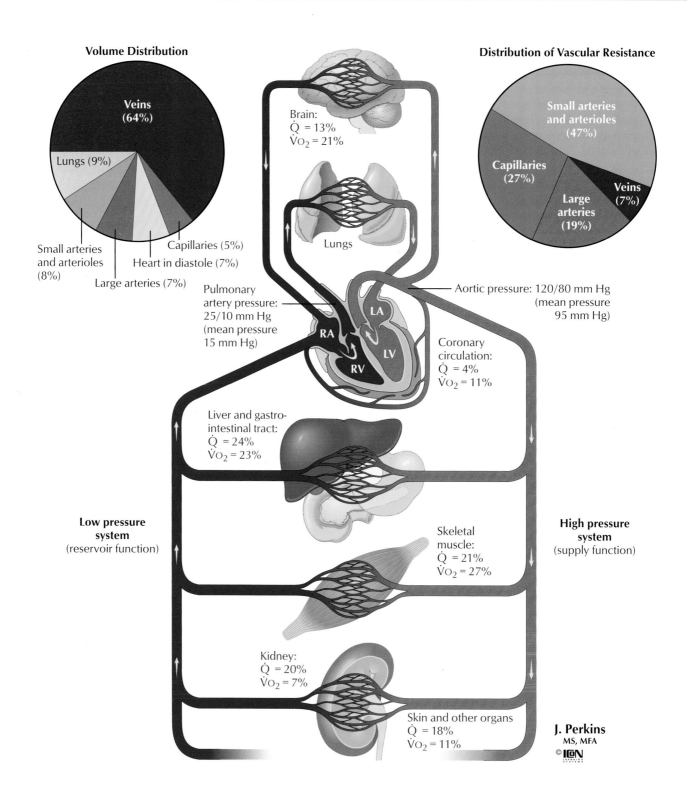

Volume Distribution

Veins (64%)

Lungs (9%)

Small arteries and arterioles (8%)

Large arteries (7%)

Heart in diastole (7%)

Capillaries (5%)

Distribution of Vascular Resistance

Small arteries and arterioles (47%)

Capillaries (27%)

Large arteries (19%)

Veins (7%)

Brain:
$\dot{Q} = 13\%$
$\dot{V}_{O_2} = 21\%$

Lungs

Pulmonary artery pressure: 25/10 mm Hg (mean pressure 15 mm Hg)

Aortic pressure: 120/80 mm Hg (mean pressure 95 mm Hg)

LA
RA
LV
RV

Coronary circulation:
$\dot{Q} = 4\%$
$\dot{V}_{O_2} = 11\%$

Liver and gastrointestinal tract:
$\dot{Q} = 24\%$
$\dot{V}_{O_2} = 23\%$

Low pressure system (reservoir function)

High pressure system (supply function)

Skeletal muscle:
$\dot{Q} = 21\%$
$\dot{V}_{O_2} = 27\%$

Kidney:
$\dot{Q} = 20\%$
$\dot{V}_{O_2} = 7\%$

Skin and other organs
$\dot{Q} = 18\%$
$\dot{V}_{O_2} = 11\%$

J. Perkins
MS, MFA
© IGN

FIGURE 4.1 CARDIOVASCULAR SYSTEM OVERVIEW

The cardiovascular system consists of the heart, which pumps blood into the pulmonary circulation for the exchange of O_2 and CO_2 and into the systemic circulation to supply all other tissues of the body. At rest, cardiac output is approximately 5 L/min in both the pulmonary and systemic circulations. The amount of blood flow ($\dot{Q}$) (as a percentage of cardiac output) and relative percentage of oxygen utilization per minute ($\dot{V}_{O_2}$) to various organ systems is shown for the resting state. The systemic circulation is arranged in a parallel fashion (brain, heart, gastrointestinal tract, etc.). Based on metabolic need and demand, both $\dot{Q}$ and $\dot{V}_{O_2}$ may be adjusted. At any one time, most of the blood volume resides in the veins (64%) and is returned to the right side of the heart. Vascular resistance is primarily a function of the small muscular arteries and arterioles.

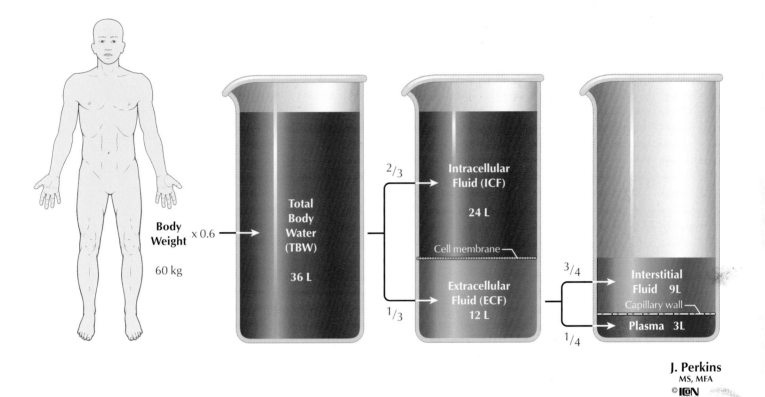

FIGURE 4.2 BODY FLUID COMPARTMENTS

Total body water (calculated for a 60-kg individual) is divided by the plasma membrane of cells into two compartments: intracellular fluid and extracellular fluid. The capillary wall subdivides the extracellular fluid into plasma (within blood vessels) and interstitial fluid. The interstitial fluid includes not only the fluid surrounding cells but also fluid in bone and dense connective tissue.

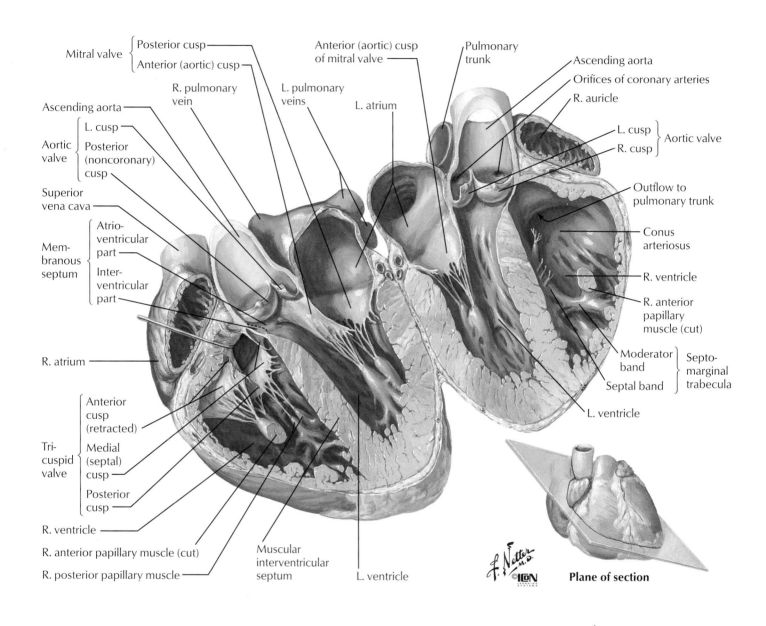

FIGURE 4.3 STRUCTURE OF HEART

This interior view of the heart shows its four chambers, valves, and septa. The right side of the heart receives blood from the systemic circulation and pumps it into the pulmonary circulation. The left side of the heart receives blood returning from the pulmonary circulation and pumps it into the systemic circulation. The work of the left ventricle is significantly greater than that of the right ventricle, and its walls are correspondingly much thicker.

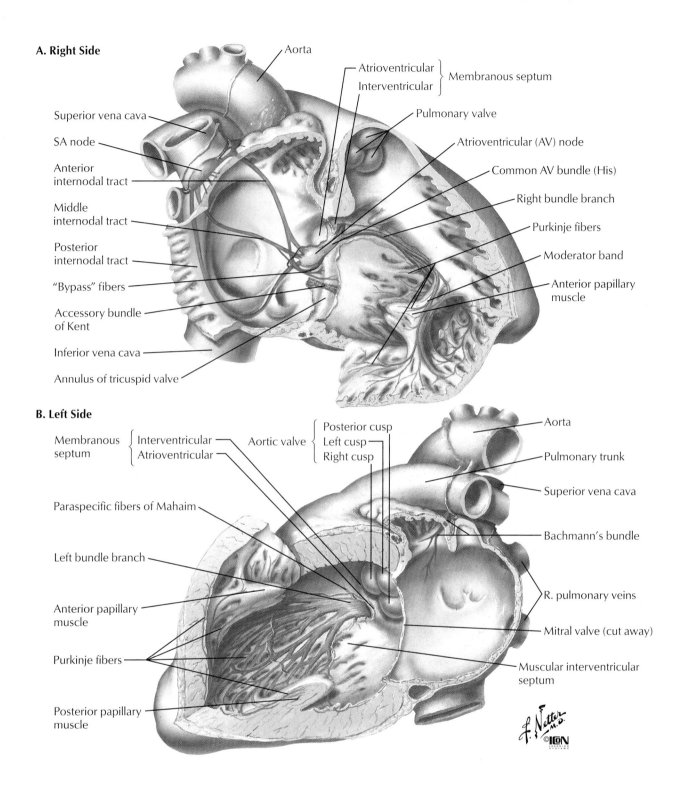

A. Right Side

- Aorta
- Atrioventricular
- Interventricular } Membranous septum
- Pulmonary valve
- Superior vena cava
- SA node
- Anterior internodal tract
- Middle internodal tract
- Posterior internodal tract
- "Bypass" fibers
- Accessory bundle of Kent
- Inferior vena cava
- Annulus of tricuspid valve
- Atrioventricular (AV) node
- Common AV bundle (His)
- Right bundle branch
- Purkinje fibers
- Moderator band
- Anterior papillary muscle

B. Left Side

- Membranous septum { Interventricular / Atrioventricular
- Aortic valve { Posterior cusp / Left cusp / Right cusp
- Aorta
- Pulmonary trunk
- Superior vena cava
- Paraspecific fibers of Mahaim
- Left bundle branch
- Anterior papillary muscle
- Purkinje fibers
- Posterior papillary muscle
- Bachmann's bundle
- R. pulmonary veins
- Mitral valve (cut away)
- Muscular interventricular septum

FIGURE 4.4   ANATOMY OF THE SPECIALIZED CONDUCTION SYSTEM

Cardiac muscle of the heart exists in two forms: the contractile myocardium and specialized conducting cells that do not contract but do spread the wave of depolarization rapidly throughout the chambers of the heart. Action potentials are initiated in the sinoatrial (SA) node, which serves as the "pacemaker" of the heart.

Impulses are conveyed to the atrioventricular (AV) node and then to the common AV bundle (of His). From here, the action potential spreads rapidly through the ventricles via the right and left bundle branches and Purkinje fiber system.

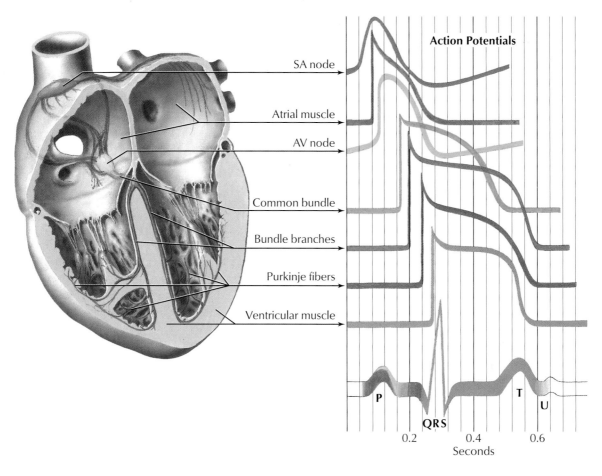

Action Potentials

SA node
Atrial muscle
AV node
Common bundle
Bundle branches
Purkinje fibers
Ventricular muscle

P
QRS
T
U

0.2   0.4   0.6
Seconds

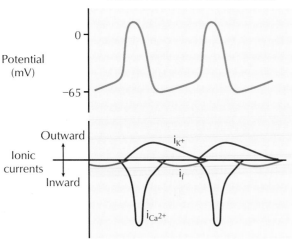

Action Potential of SA Node Cells

Potential (mV)

0
−65

Outward
Ionic currents
Inward

i_{K^+}
i_f
$i_{Ca^{2+}}$

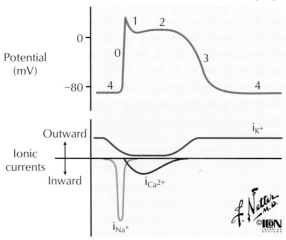

Action Potential of Ventricular Myocytes

Potential (mV)

0
−80

1   2
0   3
4   4

Outward
Ionic currents
Inward

i_{K^+}
$i_{Ca^{2+}}$
i_{Na^+}

FIGURE 4.5 ELECTRICAL ACTIVITY OF THE HEART

The normal pumping of blood through the chambers of the heart requires the precisely timed spread of action potentials through the heart's conduction system and the atrial and ventricular muscle. The rate of the heartbeat is set by spontaneously generated action potentials in the cells of the SA node. The frequency of SA node action potentials is regulated by the autonomic nervous system. Sympathetic stimulation of the SA node increases i_f (principally Na$^+$ current) and $i_{Ca^{2+}}$, which depolarizes the cell, and thereby increases the heart rate. Parasympathetic stimulation increases i_{K^+}, which hyperpolarizes the cell and thereby decreases the heart rate. The ventricular muscle action potential has a prolonged depolarization phase resulting from Ca^{2+} influx. This long plateau phase prevents tetany of cardiac muscle at very high heart rates.

Normal Sequence of Cardiac Depolarization and Repolarization and Derivation of ECG

A. Impulse origin and atrial depolarization

Impulse originates at SA node, and wave of depolarization spreads over atria, resulting in electrical vector directed downward and to left. This causes upward (positive) deflection in ECG tracing in leads I and aVF (P wave)

B. Septal depolarization

After brief delay at AV node, impulse traverses common bundle of His and right and left bundle branches and then enters interventricular septum, causing myocardial depolarization with electrical vector directed to right and downward. This results in small negative (downward) deflection in lead I (Q wave) and positive (upward) deflection in lead aVF (R wave)

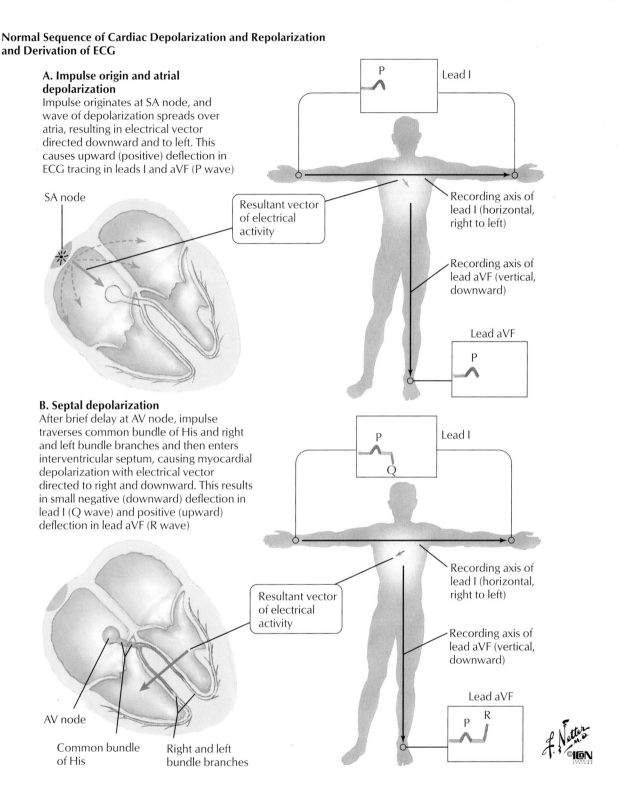

FIGURE 4.6   CARDIAC DEPOLARIZATION AND REPOLARIZATION PART 1

The elements of the electrocardiogram (ECG) are shown in the next three figures. Beginning with the SA node (pacemaker), depolarization spreads over the atria, causing an upward deflection of the ECG tracing (P wave) (panel A). The delay at the AV node ensures that the ventricles will have ample time to fill, and then the impulse passes through the bundle of His and the bundle branches of the interventricular septum. The resulting depolarization of the myocardium of the septum yields the Q wave of the ECG tracing (panel B).

Normal Sequence of Cardiac Depolarization and Repolarization and Derivation of ECG (continued)

C. Apical and early ventricular depolarization

Impulse continues along conduction system, causing depolarization of apical ventricular myocardium with electrical vector directed downward and to left. This results in large positive (upward) deflection (R wave) in lead I and extends R wave in lead aVF

D. Late ventricular depolarization

As depolarization progresses over ventricles, vector shifts to become directed superiorly as well as to left, thus extending upward R wave in lead I and causing negative (downward) deflection (S wave) in lead aVF

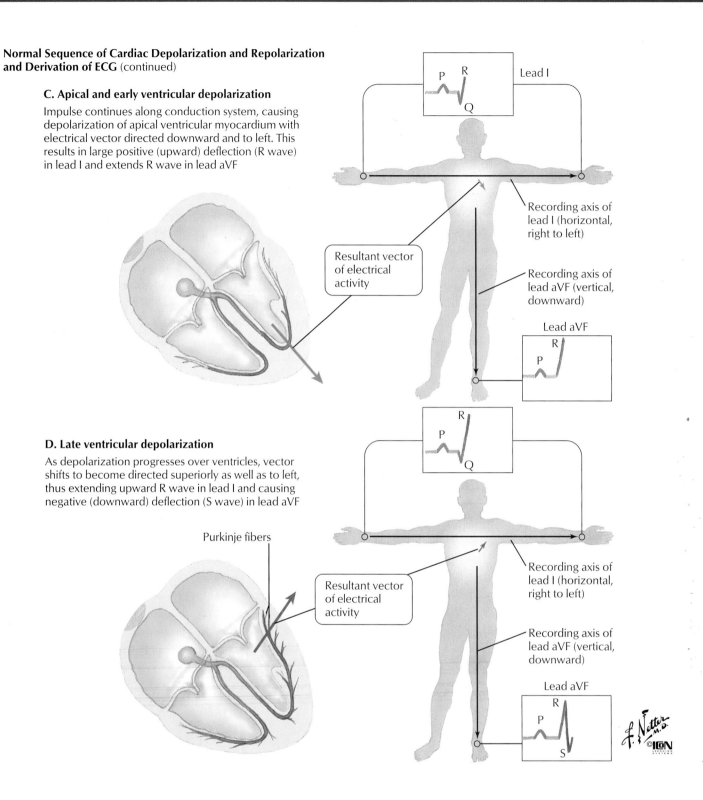

FIGURE 4.7   CARDIAC DEPOLARIZATION AND REPOLARIZATION PART 2

ECG continued. As the apex of the ventricles contracts, a large upward positive deflection of the tracing yields the R wave of the ECG (panel C). Then the wave of depolarization spreads through the ventricular walls, causing the S wave of the ECG tracing (panel D).

Normal Sequence of Cardiac Depolarization and Repolarization and Derivation of ECG (continued)

E. Repolarization

When heart is fully depolarized, there is no electrical activity for brief period (ST segment). Then repolarization begins from endocardium to epicardium, producing electrical vector directed downward and to left, causing upward (positive) deflection in both leads I and aVF (T waves). A period of no electrical activity follows, with tracing at baseline until next impulse originates at SA node

F. Summary of cardiac electrical activity

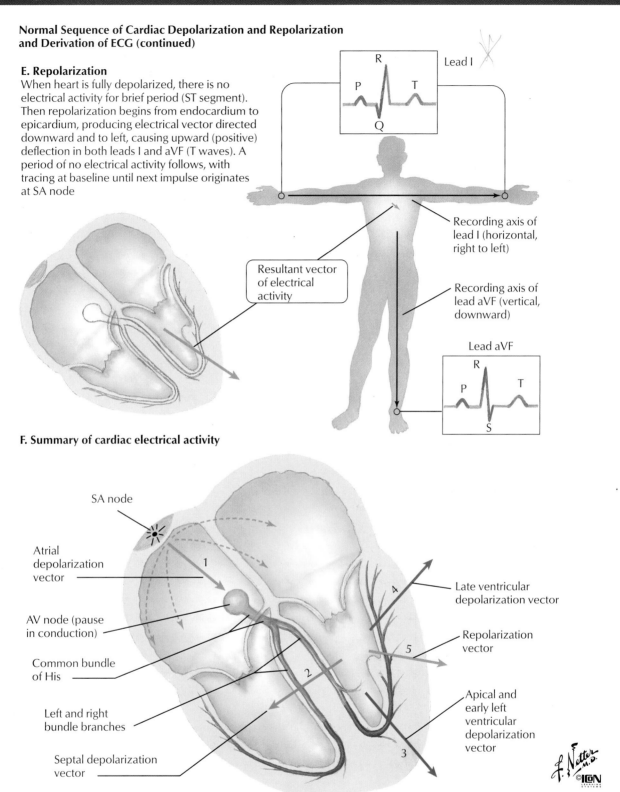

Lead I

Resultant vector of electrical activity

Recording axis of lead I (horizontal, right to left)

Recording axis of lead aVF (vertical, downward)

Lead aVF

SA node

Atrial depolarization vector

AV node (pause in conduction)

Common bundle of His

Left and right bundle branches

Septal depolarization vector

Late ventricular depolarization vector

Repolarization vector

Apical and early left ventricular depolarization vector

FIGURE 4.8   CARDIAC DEPOLARIZATION AND REPOLARIZATION PART 3

ECG continued. Once fully depolarized, electrical activity ceases briefly (the ST segment of the tracing), and then repolarization begins, moving from the inner endocardium to the outer epi-cardium, generating the T wave of the ECG tracing (panel E). Panel F summarizes the sequence of events in myocardial depolarization and repolarization.

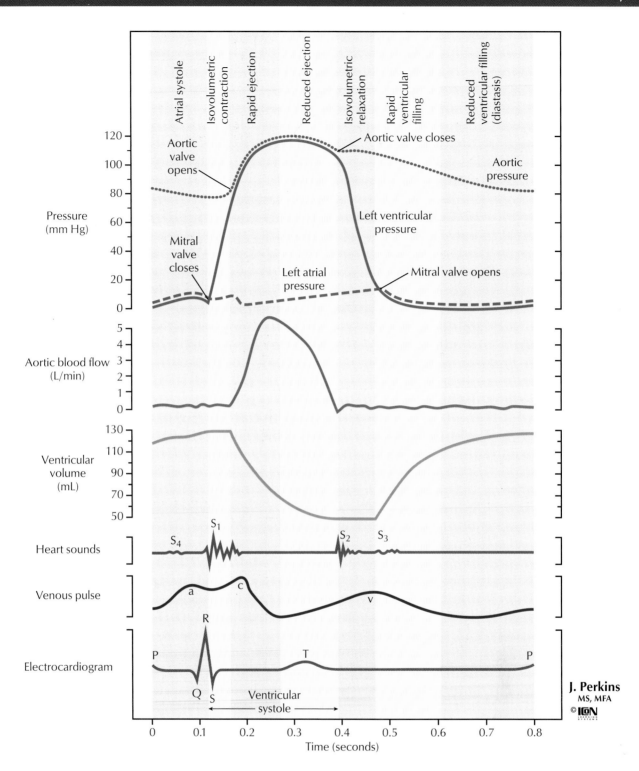

FIGURE 4.9 CARDIAC CYCLE

The cardiac cycle represents one complete sequence of atrial and ventricular contraction and relaxation. Depicted here are the key electrical and hemodynamic events associated with a single cycle. Changes in left atrial, ventricular, and aortic pressure; aortic blood flow; ventricular volume; heart sounds; jugular venous pressure; and the ECG are shown. The S_1 heart sound results from the closing of the mitral and tricuspid valves, whereas the S_2 heart sound results from the closing of the aortic and pulmonic valves. Both S_3 and S_4 are sounds associated with filling of the ventricles. They are nor-mally difficult to hear in healthy adults. S_3 is heard in healthy children and in states of high cardiac output. S_4 is associated with ventricular filling during atrial contraction. The components of the jugular venous pulse are the *a* wave, caused by right atrial contraction; the *c* wave, which results from bulging of the tricuspid valve into right atrium during right ventricular contraction; and the *v* wave, resulting from increased right atrial volume (and pressure) as venous blood fills this chamber before the opening of the tricuspid valve. The components of the ECG are described in Figures 4.6 to 4.8.

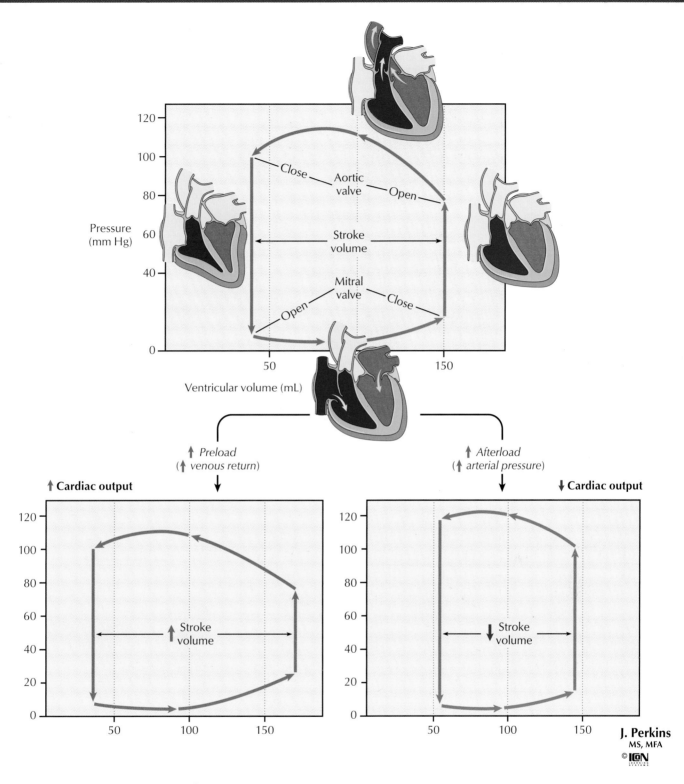

FIGURE 4.10   PRESSURE-VOLUME LOOP

Cardiac output is the volume of blood pumped by the heart each minute. In the steady state the output from both the right and left ventricles is the same. The pressure-volume loop for the left ventricle is depicted here. The cardiac output is calculated as:

Cardiac output = Heart rate × Stroke volume

where:

Stroke volume = End-diastolic volume − End-systolic volume

Increases in venous return (increased preload) increase the stroke volume and thus cardiac output. Increases in arterial pressure (increased afterload) decrease stroke volume and thus cardiac output (lower panel).

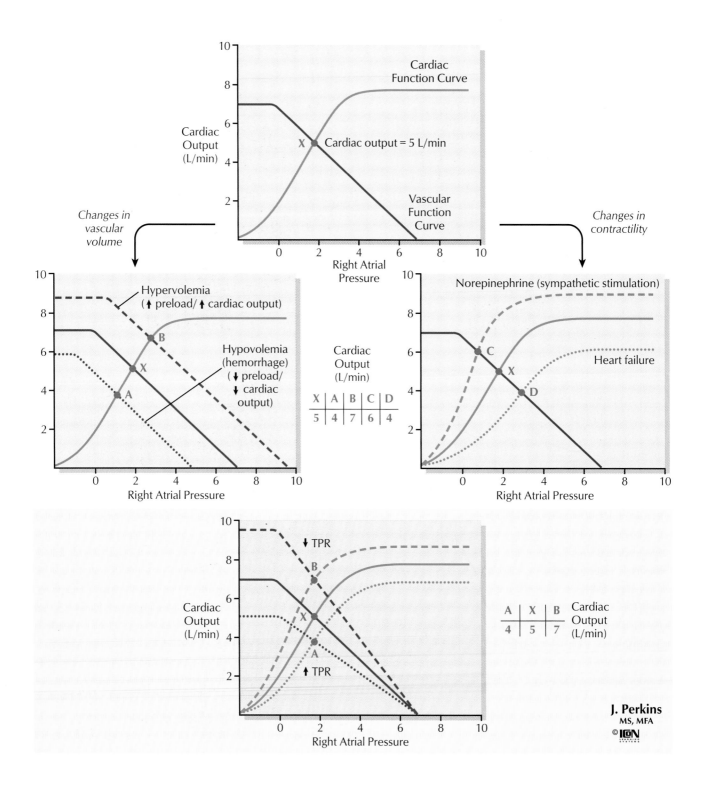

FIGURE 4.11   CARDIAC AND VASCULAR FUNCTION CURVES

The heart and blood vessels interact with each other to determine cardiac output. Depicted here are a series of vascular and cardiac function curves that illustrate this interaction. Changes in right atrial pressure affect venous return. Changes in vascular volume affect the vascular function curves, and changes in cardiac contractility affect the cardiac function curve. Changes in total peripheral resistance (TPR) affect both the vascular and cardiac function curves.

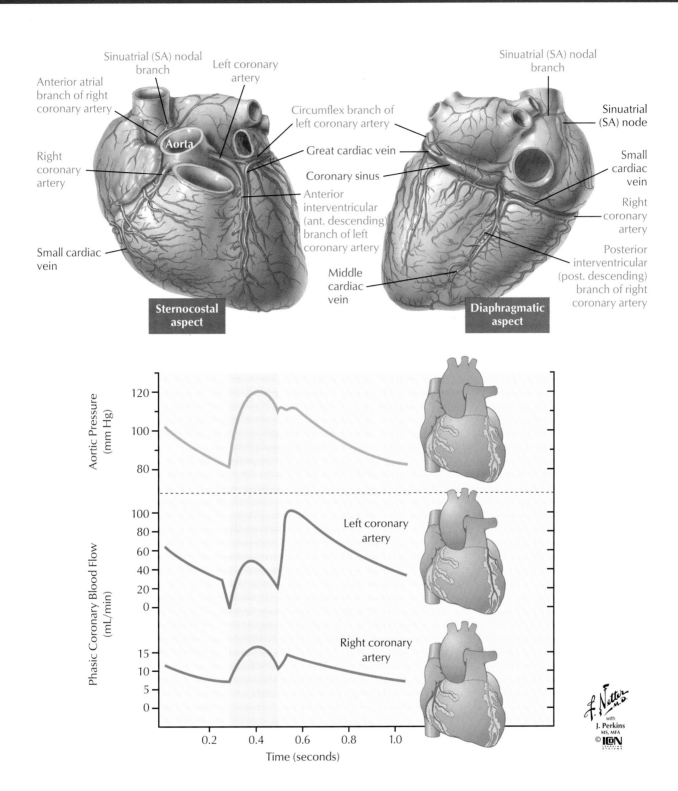

FIGURE 4.12 CORONARY CIRCULATION

The coronary arteries come off the aorta just above the aortic valve. Coronary blood flow varies with aortic pressure but is influenced by physical factors (compression of the vessels during contraction of the heart) and by metabolic factors released from the myocytes. Numerous metabolic factors have been implicated in the regulation of coronary blood flow (e.g., H^+, CO_2, decreased O_2, K^+, lactic acid, nitric oxide, adenosine). Of these factors, adenosine seems to be the most important. Thus, when cardiac work demand increases, adenosine released by the myocytes leads to vasodilation and thereby increased coronary blood flow.

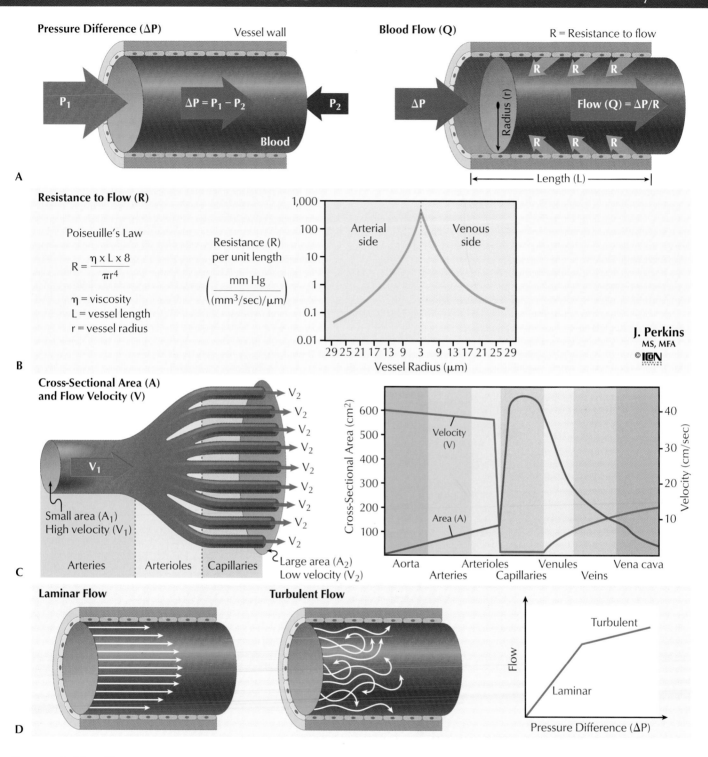

Pressure Difference (ΔP)

Vessel wall

P_1

$\Delta P = P_1 - P_2$

P_2

Blood

A

Blood Flow (Q)

R = Resistance to flow

ΔP

Radius (r)

Flow (Q) = ΔP/R

Length (L)

Resistance to Flow (R)

Poiseuille's Law

$$R = \frac{\eta \times L \times 8}{\pi r^4}$$

η = viscosity
L = vessel length
r = vessel radius

Resistance (R) per unit length

$$\left(\frac{mm\ Hg}{(mm^3/sec)/\mu m}\right)$$

Arterial side

Venous side

Vessel Radius (μm)

J. Perkins
MS, MFA

B

Cross-Sectional Area (A) and Flow Velocity (V)

V_1

V_2

Small area (A_1)
High velocity (V_1)

Large area (A_2)
Low velocity (V_2)

Arteries   Arterioles   Capillaries

Cross-Sectional Area (cm²)

Velocity (V)

Area (A)

Velocity (cm/sec)

Aorta   Arterioles   Venules   Vena cava
Arteries   Capillaries   Veins

C

Laminar Flow

Turbulent Flow

Turbulent

Laminar

Flow

Pressure Difference (ΔP)

D

FIGURE 4.13   HEMODYNAMICS

Panel A: The flow of blood flow through a vessel (Q) depends on the pressure difference (ΔP) and the resistance to flow (R). In the systemic circulation, ΔP = aortic pressure − right atrial pressure, and R = the total peripheral resistance (TPR). *Panel B:* As described by Poiseuille's law, the most important factor determining resistance to blood flow is the radius of the vessel. The small arterioles and capillaries have the highest resistance. Because of their ability to regulate their tone, the small arterioles are the most important vessels involved in regulating the TPR. *Panel C:* As blood flows from the aorta it courses through an increasingly branched arterial system. This branching increases the total cross-sectional area through which the blood flows and reduces the velocity of this flow (V = Q/A). The reduced flow velocity in the capillaries facilitates the exchange of fluids and nutrients across the capillary wall by allowing sufficient time for diffusion to occur. *Panel D:* Normally, blood flow through most of the vascular system is laminar. The exception is at the root of the aorta. However, in pathological conditions (e.g., lesions of the heart valves, narrowing or partial blockage of vessels), turbulent flow occurs and can be heard with the stethoscope as murmurs (in the heart) or bruits (in vessels). Laminar flow reduces the pressure gradient needed to propel the blood through the vessel.

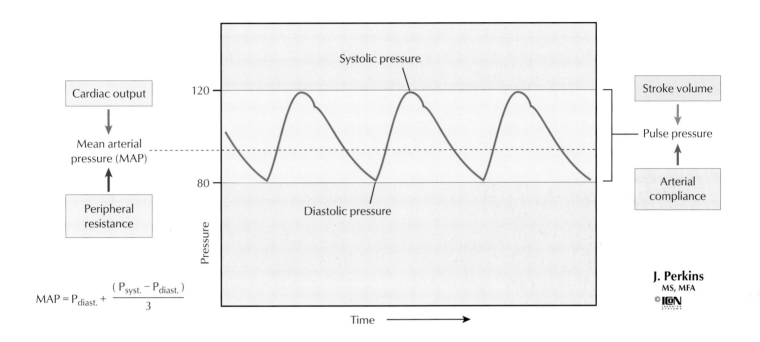

FIGURE 4.14   ARTERIAL PRESSURE

The mean arterial pressure (MAP) is the average pressure in the arteries averaged over time. It is determined by the cardiac output (CO) and the total peripheral resistance (TPR) as: MAP = CO × TPR. As described in Figure 4.10, CO is determined by the stroke volume (SV) and heart rate (HR) as: CO = SV × HR. Blood volume is an important determinant of SV. The sympathetic nervous system and a number of hormones (see Figure 4.15) determine vascular resistance. As a result of the heart's rhythmic pumping, the arterial pressure is pulsatile. The pulse pressure depends on the SV (large SV increases the pulse pressure) and the compliance of the arterial wall (decreased compliance increases pulse pressure). With normal aging, compliance of the arterial wall increases and results in an increase in the pulse pressure.

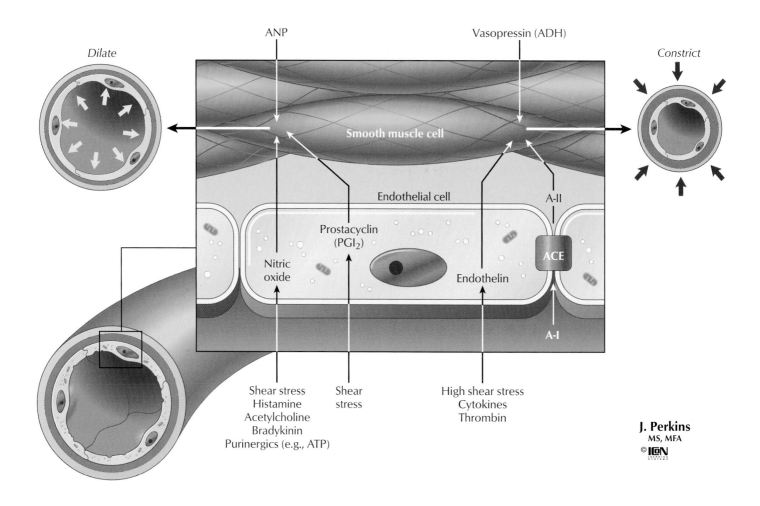

FIGURE 4.15 CONTROL OF ARTERIOLAR TONE

Small arterioles are the major determinants of the resistance of the vascular system. Release of norepinephrine by sympathetic nerves contributes to the resting tone of the smooth muscle cell and, with increased sympathetic firing, further increases tone. Circulating hormones such as atrial natriuretic peptide (ANP), angiotensin II (A-II) and vasopressin (ADH) also act on the arterial smooth muscle cells to alter their tone. Substances produced by the endothelial cells in response to a host of factors (e.g., sheer stress due to blood flowing through the vessel and acetylcholine released from parasympathetic nerves) act on the adjacent arterial smooth muscle cells to modulate their tone. The surface of the endothelial cell also contains angiotensin-converting enzyme (ACE), which is necessary to convert the inactive angiotensin I (A-I) molecule to its active form A-II.

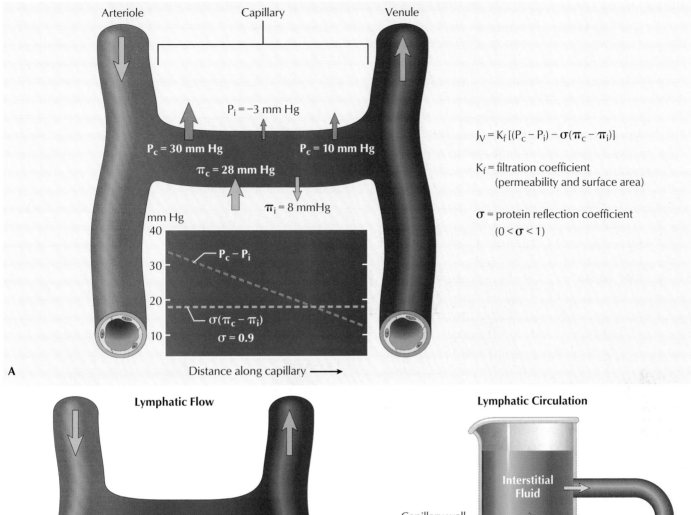

$$J_V = K_f [(P_c - P_i) - \sigma(\pi_c - \pi_i)]$$

K_f = filtration coefficient
(permeability and surface area)

σ = protein reflection coefficient
$(0 < \sigma < 1)$

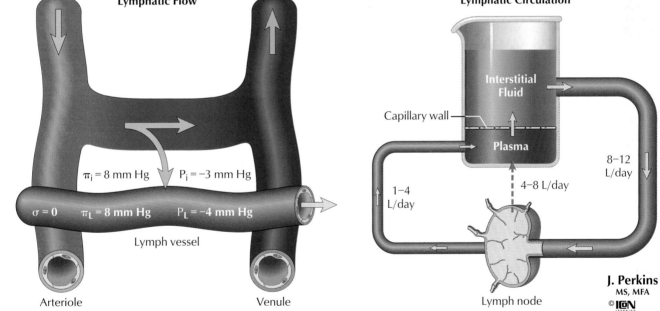

FIGURE 4.16 MICROCIRCULATION

Exchange of O_2, CO_2, nutrients, cellular metabolites, and fluid occurs across the capillary wall by both diffusion and bulk flow. As shown in *panel A*, bulk flow of fluid across the capillary wall is driven by the Starling forces (i.e., hydrostatic pressure — P and oncotic pressure generated by proteins — Π). Hydrostatic pressure results from the pumping of blood by the heart, as well as the effect of gravity on the column of blood in a vessel. Oncotic pressure represents the osmotic pressure generated by proteins. In addition to these Starling forces, the volume of fluid moving across the capillary wall depends on the filtration coefficient (K_f), which reflects the intrinsic permeability of the wall and its surface area. The proteins in plasma and interstitial fluid can exert an osmotic pressure only if they do not readily cross the capillary wall. The ease with which proteins cross the wall is expressed by the reflection coefficient (σ). Proteins do not easily cross the wall in skeletal muscle capillaries ($\sigma = 0.9$) and therefore play an important role in fluid movement. However, liver capillaries (termed sinusoids) are highly permeable to proteins. As a result, $\sigma = 0$, and the protein oncotic pressure does not contribute to the movement of fluid across the sinusoid wall (i.e., fluid movement in the liver sinusoid occurs only by hydrostatic pressure). *Panel B:* In most capillary beds there is net movement of fluid out of the capillary into the interstitium. This fluid is carried away by lymphatic vessels and returned to the vascular compartment either at lymph nodes or by the thoracic and right lymphatic ducts.

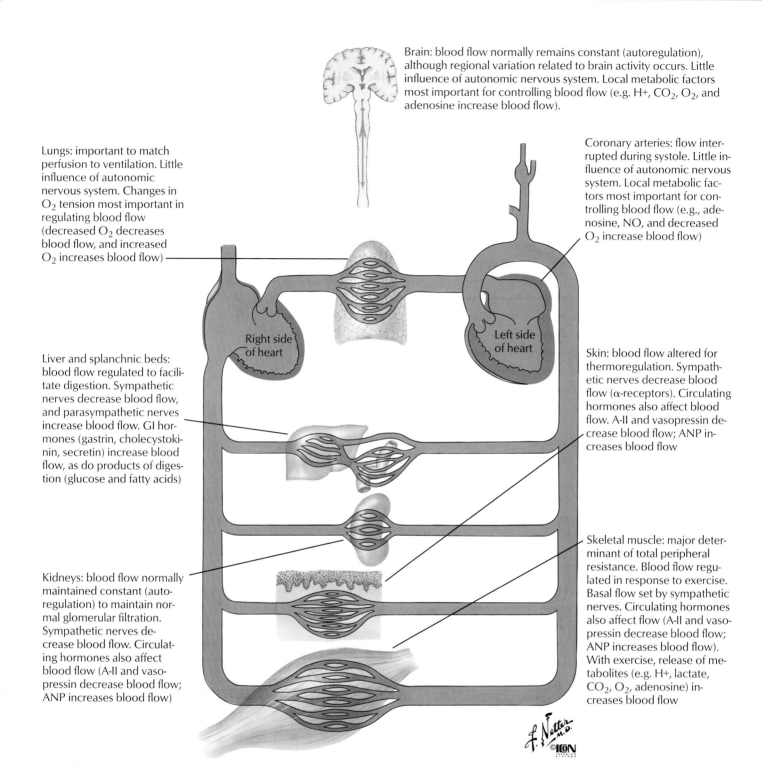

Brain: blood flow normally remains constant (autoregulation), although regional variation related to brain activity occurs. Little influence of autonomic nervous system. Local metabolic factors most important for controlling blood flow (e.g. H+, CO_2, O_2, and adenosine increase blood flow).

Lungs: important to match perfusion to ventilation. Little influence of autonomic nervous system. Changes in O_2 tension most important in regulating blood flow (decreased O_2 decreases blood flow, and increased O_2 increases blood flow)

Coronary arteries: flow interrupted during systole. Little influence of autonomic nervous system. Local metabolic factors most important for controlling blood flow (e.g., adenosine, NO, and decreased O_2 increase blood flow)

Liver and splanchnic beds: blood flow regulated to facilitate digestion. Sympathetic nerves decrease blood flow, and parasympathetic nerves increase blood flow. GI hormones (gastrin, cholecystokinin, secretin) increase blood flow, as do products of digestion (glucose and fatty acids)

Right side of heart

Left side of heart

Skin: blood flow altered for thermoregulation. Sympathetic nerves decrease blood flow (α-receptors). Circulating hormones also affect blood flow. A-II and vasopressin decrease blood flow; ANP increases blood flow

Kidneys: blood flow normally maintained constant (autoregulation) to maintain normal glomerular filtration. Sympathetic nerves decrease blood flow. Circulating hormones also affect blood flow (A-II and vasopressin decrease blood flow; ANP increases blood flow)

Skeletal muscle: major determinant of total peripheral resistance. Blood flow regulated in response to exercise. Basal flow set by sympathetic nerves. Circulating hormones also affect flow (A-II and vasopressin decrease blood flow; ANP increases blood flow). With exercise, release of metabolites (e.g. H+, lactate, CO_2, O_2, adenosine) increases blood flow

FIGURE 4.17 CIRCULATION TO SPECIAL REGIONS

Blood flow to different vascular beds is regulated by a number of factors and in response to the physiological demands of the tissues.

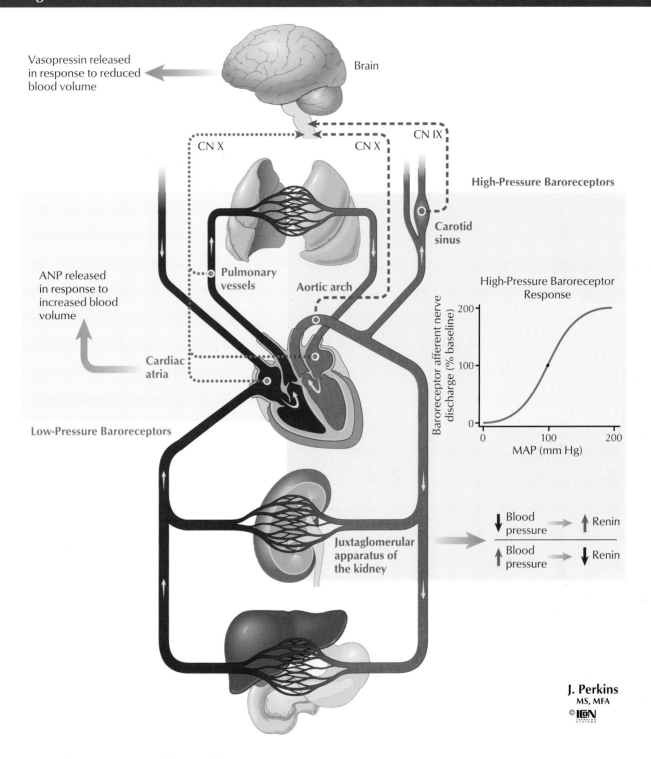

FIGURE 4.18   MONITORING OF BLOOD PRESSURE

The body has a complex system to monitor and regulate blood pressure (BP). This system is critically important for the maintenance of BP during all aspects of daily life (e.g., rising from a sitting to a standing position or during exercise), as well as during abnormal conditions (e.g., excessive fluid loss in a hot environment or hemorrhage). Pressure sensors (termed baroreceptors) are located in the high-pressure (arterial) and low-pressure (venous) sides of the circulatory system. High-pressure baroreceptors in the aortic arch and carotid sinus monitor arterial BP and send signals to the brainstem in the vagus (CN X) and glossopharyngeal (CN IX) nerves. These signals result in alterations in sympathetic nerve activity (not shown). The afferent arterioles of the juxtaglomerular apparatus are also high-pressure baroreceptors.

They respond to changes in arterial BP by varying the secretion of the proteolytic enzyme renin. As described in Figure 6.12, renin results in the production of angiotensin II, a potent vasoconstrictor (see Figure 4.15). Low-pressure baroreceptors are found in the large pulmonary vessels and the atria of the heart. By their location, they respond primarily to changes in blood volume. These baroreceptors send signals to the brain in the vagus nerve (CN X), which, in addition to altering sympathetic nerve activity, cause the release of vasopressin (ADH). When stretched (i.e., increased blood volume) the atria also secrete the hormone atrial natriuretic peptide (ANP), which increases the excretion of NaCl and water by the kidneys (see Figure 4.20) and decreases arterial tone (see Figure 4.15).

83

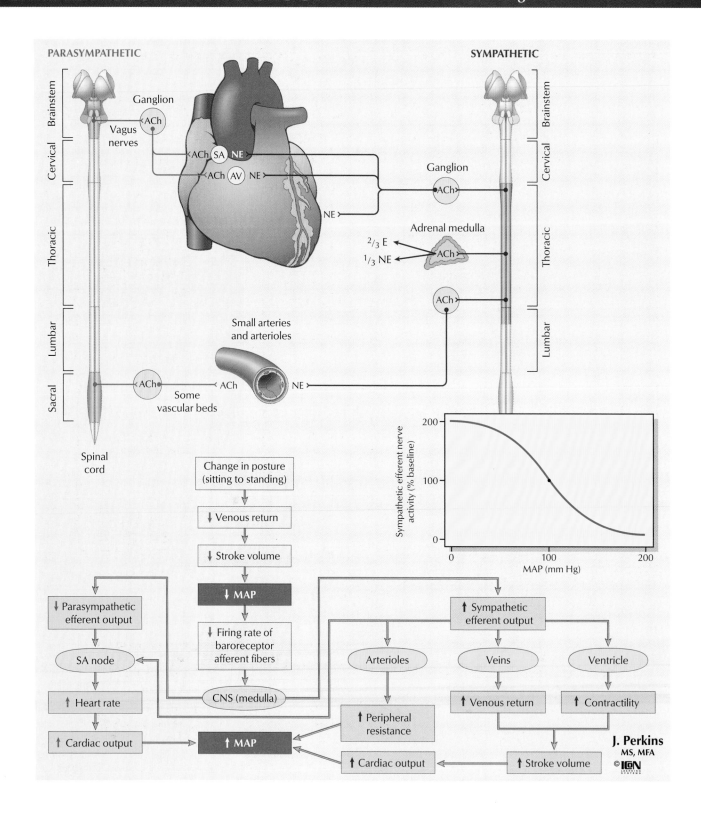

FIGURE 4.19   SHORT-TERM RESPONSE TO CHANGES IN BLOOD PRESSURE

The autonomic nervous system is primarily involved in maintaining blood pressure on a second-by-second basis. This is illustrated for a change in posture. *ACh*, Acetylcholine; *E*, epinephrine; *NE*, norepinephrine; *MAP*, mean arterial pressure.

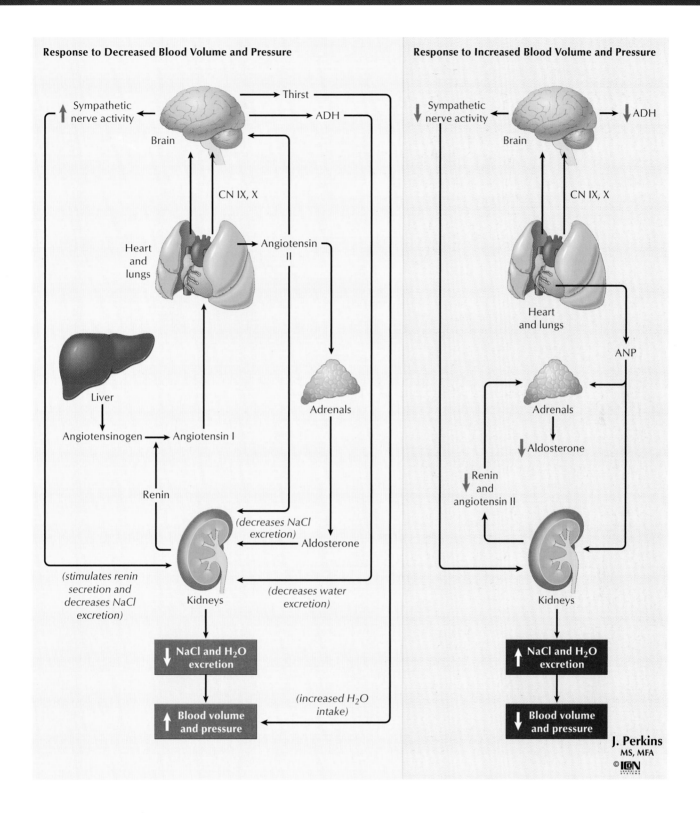

Response to Decreased Blood Volume and Pressure

Response to Increased Blood Volume and Pressure

↑ Sympathetic nerve activity

Thirst

ADH

Brain

CN IX, X

Heart and lungs

Angiotensin II

Liver

Angiotensinogen → Angiotensin I

Renin

Adrenals

(decreases NaCl excretion)

Aldosterone

(stimulates renin secretion and decreases NaCl excretion)

Kidneys

(decreases water excretion)

↓ NaCl and H₂O excretion

↑ Blood volume and pressure

(increased H₂O intake)

↓ Sympathetic nerve activity

↓ ADH

Brain

CN IX, X

Heart and lungs

ANP

Adrenals

↓ Aldosterone

↓ Renin and angiotensin II

Kidneys

↑ NaCl and H₂O excretion

↓ Blood volume and pressure

J. Perkins
MS, MFA
© ICON

FIGURE 4.20 LONG-TERM RESPONSE TO CHANGES IN BLOOD VOLUME AND PRESSURE

When blood volume (and pressure) changes, the kidneys respond by either retaining NaCl and water or excreting NaCl and water in order to restore blood volume to its normal value. With increased sympathetic nerve activity, norepinephrine and epinephrine secre-tion by the adrenal medulla will be stimulated (not shown). These circulating catecholamines will also act on the kidney to reduce NaCl excretion.

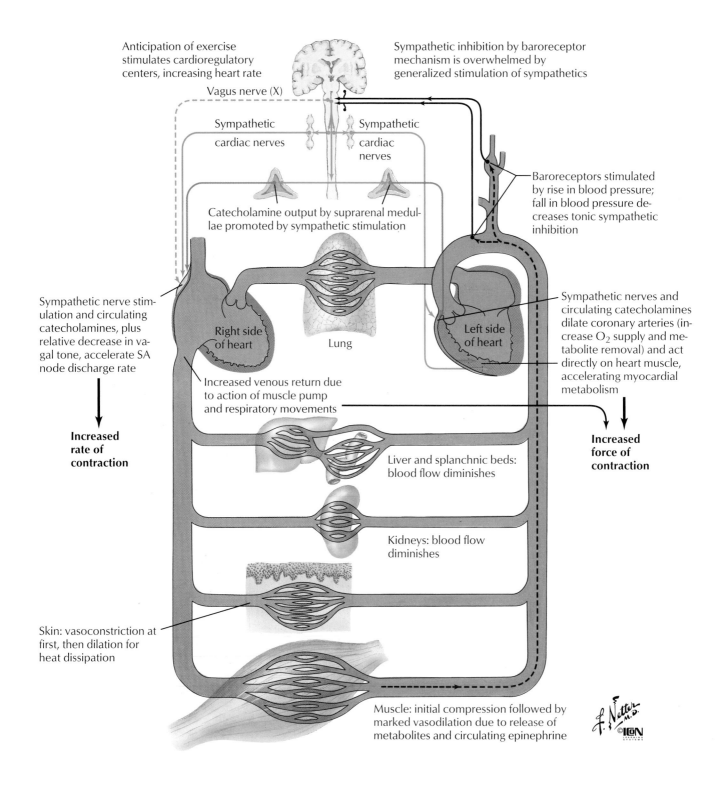

Anticipation of exercise stimulates cardioregulatory centers, increasing heart rate

Vagus nerve (X)

Sympathetic inhibition by baroreceptor mechanism is overwhelmed by generalized stimulation of sympathetics

Sympathetic cardiac nerves

Sympathetic cardiac nerves

Baroreceptors stimulated by rise in blood pressure; fall in blood pressure decreases tonic sympathetic inhibition

Catecholamine output by suprarenal medullae promoted by sympathetic stimulation

Sympathetic nerve stimulation and circulating catecholamines, plus relative decrease in vagal tone, accelerate SA node discharge rate

Right side of heart

Lung

Left side of heart

Sympathetic nerves and circulating catecholamines dilate coronary arteries (increase O_2 supply and metabolite removal) and act directly on heart muscle, accelerating myocardial metabolism

Increased rate of contraction

Increased venous return due to action of muscle pump and respiratory movements

Increased force of contraction

Liver and splanchnic beds: blood flow diminishes

Kidneys: blood flow diminishes

Skin: vasoconstriction at first, then dilation for heat dissipation

Muscle: initial compression followed by marked vasodilation due to release of metabolites and circulating epinephrine

FIGURE 4.21 CIRCULATORY RESPONSE TO EXERCISE

This figure summarizes the integrated neural and chemical effects of exercise on the cardiovascular system. Neural effects are mediated centrally (by the autonomic nervous system), whereas the chemical effects are mediated locally by the release of vasoactive metabolites and the effects of circulating catecholamines (e.g., epinephrine).

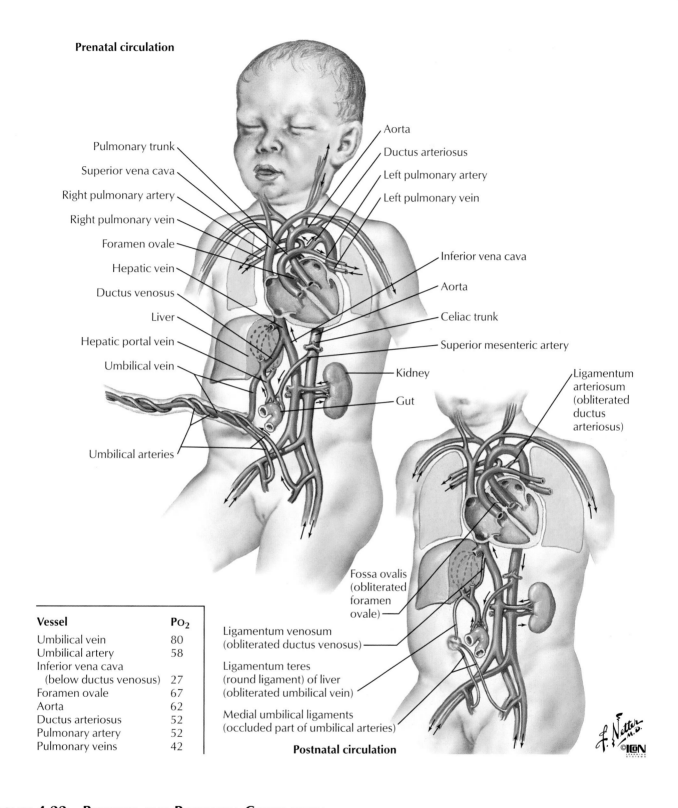

Prenatal circulation

Postnatal circulation

Vessel	PO$_2$
Umbilical vein	80
Umbilical artery	58
Inferior vena cava	
(below ductus venosus)	27
Foramen ovale	67
Aorta	62
Ductus arteriosus	52
Pulmonary artery	52
Pulmonary veins	42

FIGURE 4.22   PRENATAL AND POSTNATAL CIRCULATION

This figure summarizes prenatal and postnatal circulation. Postnatally, blood no longer passes through the placenta but does perfuse the lungs. Consequently, prenatal shunts that delivered blood to the placenta and back to the fetus (umbilical arteries and umbilical vein) become ligaments. Likewise, shunts bypassing the liver (ductus venosus), the right ventricle (foramen ovale), and the pulmonary circulation (ductus arteriosus) also close, providing for the pulmonary and systemic circulations that characterize the normal postnatal pattern. Values on the lower left represent relative percentages of O$_2$ saturation of the blood at various points along the fetal circulation.

Chapter 5 Respiratory Physiology

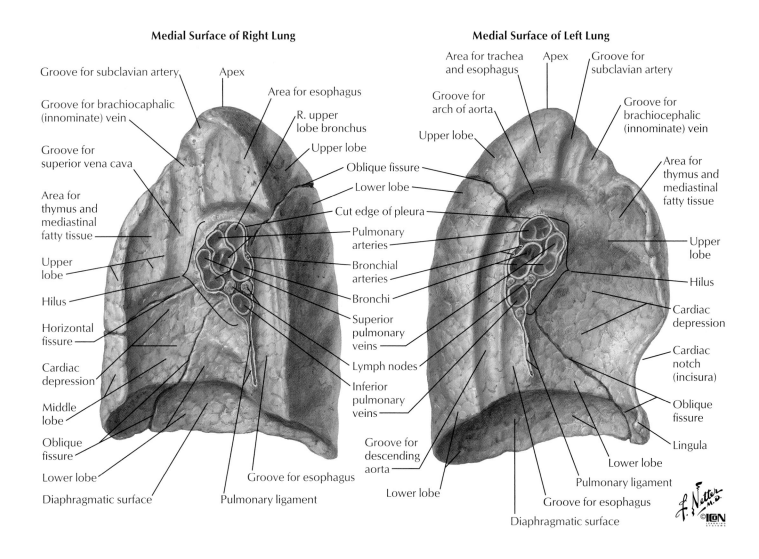

Medial Surface of Right Lung

Groove for subclavian artery
Apex
Area for esophagus
R. upper lobe bronchus
Upper lobe
Oblique fissure
Lower lobe
Cut edge of pleura
Pulmonary arteries
Bronchial arteries
Bronchi
Superior pulmonary veins
Lymph nodes
Inferior pulmonary veins

Groove for brachiocaphalic (innominate) vein
Groove for superior vena cava
Area for thymus and mediastinal fatty tissue
Upper lobe
Hilus
Horizontal fissure
Cardiac depression
Middle lobe
Oblique fissure
Lower lobe
Diaphragmatic surface
Groove for esophagus
Pulmonary ligament

Medial Surface of Left Lung

Area for trachea and esophagus
Apex
Groove for subclavian artery
Groove for arch of aorta
Upper lobe
Groove for brachiocephalic (innominate) vein
Area for thymus and mediastinal fatty tissue
Upper lobe
Hilus
Cardiac depression
Cardiac notch (incisura)
Oblique fissure
Lingula
Lower lobe
Pulmonary ligament
Groove for descending aorta
Lower lobe
Groove for esophagus
Diaphragmatic surface

FIGURE 5.1   MEDIAL SURFACE OF THE LUNGS

Breathing, or ventilation of the lungs, is an automatic, usually rhythmic, and centrally controlled process. The right lung has three lobes, and the left lung has two lobes, with the bronchi, pulmonary vessels, nerves, and lymphatics entering or leaving each lung at the hilum, which is situated on the medial aspect of the lung. The trachea bifurcates into primary bronchi, which then enter the lobes of the lung and further subdivide into smaller and smaller segments (bronchioles and ultimately alveolar ducts and sacs).

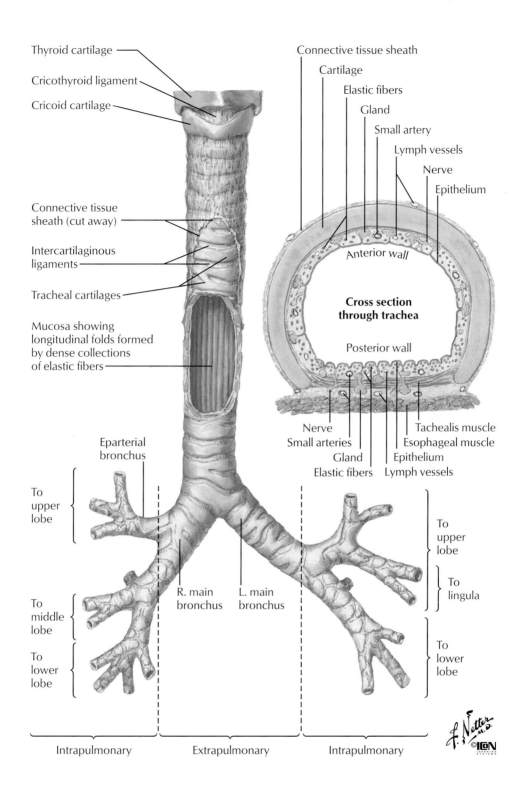

Thyroid cartilage

Cricothyroid ligament

Cricoid cartilage

Connective tissue sheath (cut away)

Intercartilaginous ligaments

Tracheal cartilages

Mucosa showing longitudinal folds formed by dense collections of elastic fibers

Connective tissue sheath

Cartilage

Elastic fibers

Gland

Small artery

Lymph vessels

Nerve

Epithelium

Anterior wall

Cross section through trachea

Posterior wall

Nerve

Small arteries

Gland

Elastic fibers

Tachealis muscle

Esophageal muscle

Epithelium

Lymph vessels

Eparterial bronchus

To upper lobe

To middle lobe

To lower lobe

R. main bronchus

L. main bronchus

To upper lobe

To lingula

To lower lobe

Intrapulmonary　　Extrapulmonary　　Intrapulmonary

FIGURE 5.2　STRUCTURE OF THE TRACHEA AND MAJOR BRONCHI

The major conducting airways to the lungs include the cartilaginous trachea, the right and left main bronchus, and the intrapulmonary bronchi passing through the lung parenchyma. With each subsequent branching, the conducting airways become smaller and smaller in diameter (see Figure 5.3), eventually losing their cartilaginous plates.

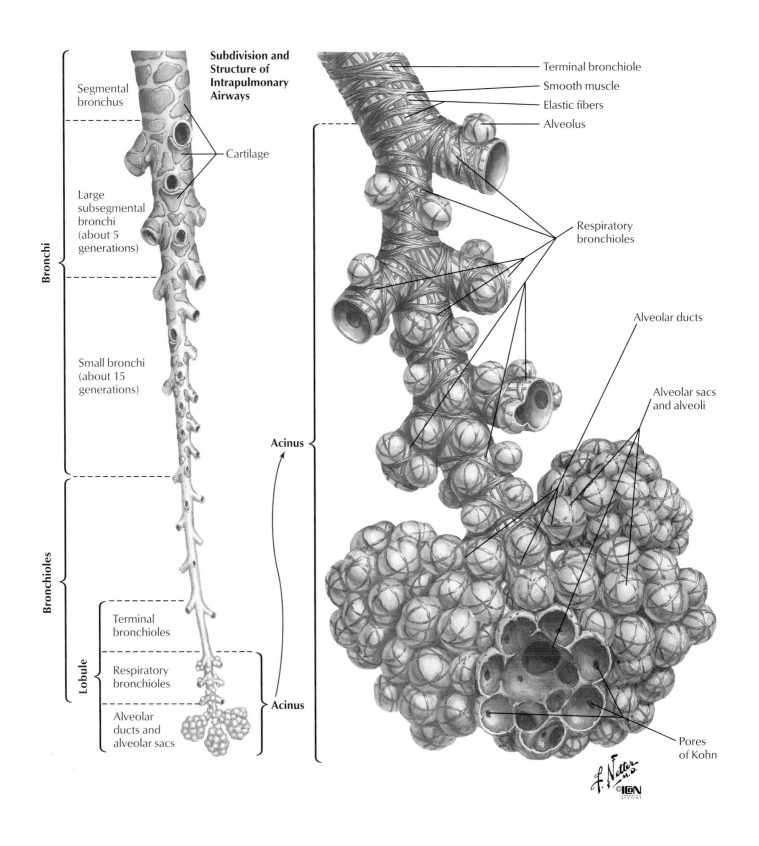

Subdivision and Structure of Intrapulmonary Airways

Segmental bronchus

Cartilage

Large subsegmental bronchi (about 5 generations)

Small bronchi (about 15 generations)

Acinus

Terminal bronchioles

Respiratory bronchioles

Alveolar ducts and alveolar sacs

Acinus

Bronchi

Bronchioles

Lobule

Terminal bronchiole

Smooth muscle

Elastic fibers

Alveolus

Respiratory bronchioles

Alveolar ducts

Alveolar sacs and alveoli

Pores of Kohn

FIGURE 5.3   INTRAPULMONARY AIRWAYS

As air enters the trachea during inspiration, it will pass through as few as 10 or as many as 23 generations, or branchings, on its journey to alveoli. The initial bronchi constitute the conducting zone and are incapable of gas exchange. Bronchioles represent a transitional zone with some alveoli, and the terminal bronchioles are lined with alveolar ducts and sacs, representing the respiratory zone.

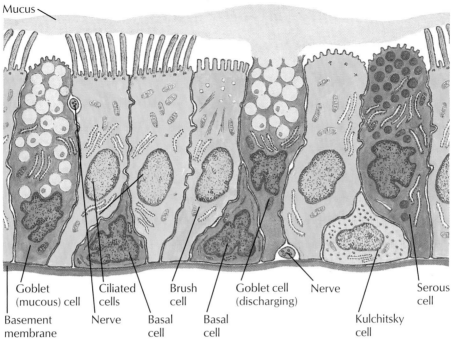

Mucus

Goblet (mucous) cell | Ciliated cells | Brush cell | Goblet cell (discharging) | Nerve | Serous cell

Basement membrane | Nerve | Basal cell | Basal cell | Kulchitsky cell

Trachea and large bronchi. Ciliated and goblet cells predominant, with some serous cells and occasional brush cells and Clara cells. Numerous basal cells and occasional Kulchitsky cells are present

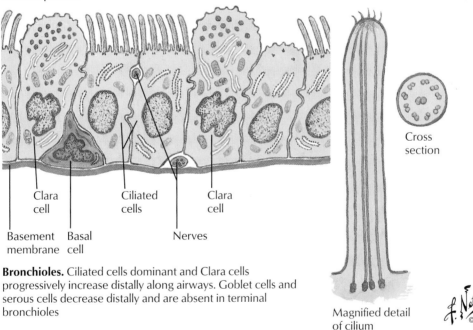

Clara cell | Ciliated cells | Clara cell

Basement membrane | Basal cell | Nerves

Cross section

Bronchioles. Ciliated cells dominant and Clara cells progressively increase distally along airways. Goblet cells and serous cells decrease distally and are absent in terminal bronchioles

Magnified detail of cilium

FIGURE 5.4 ULTRASTRUCTURE OF TRACHEAL, BRONCHIAL, AND BRONCHIOLAR EPITHELIUM

The respiratory airways are lined by a pseudostratified, ciliated columnar epithelium. In smaller airways the epithelium may become low columnar or simple cuboidal. The ciliated cells constitute approximately 30% of the total cell population. Goblet cells (30% of cell population) secrete mucus that coats the epithelial cells. This mucous coating protects the epithelial cells from desiccation and traps inhaled particulates that are then transported up the airways and out of the lungs by the ciliated cells—a process termed mucociliary transport. Basal cells (30% of cell population) are stem cells that give rise to the goblet, ciliated, and brush cells.

The function of brush cells (3% of cell population) is not resolved. They may represent goblet cells that have released their contents, or they may have a sensory role. The Kulchitsky cells (3% of cell population) secrete a number of paracrine factors that likely regulate the function of nearby cells. They are part of the bodies diffuse neuroendocrine system (DNES). Clara cells secrete a surfactant-like material that reduces surface tension of the bronchioles. They may also degrade inhaled toxins. The function of the secretory product of the serous cells is not known.

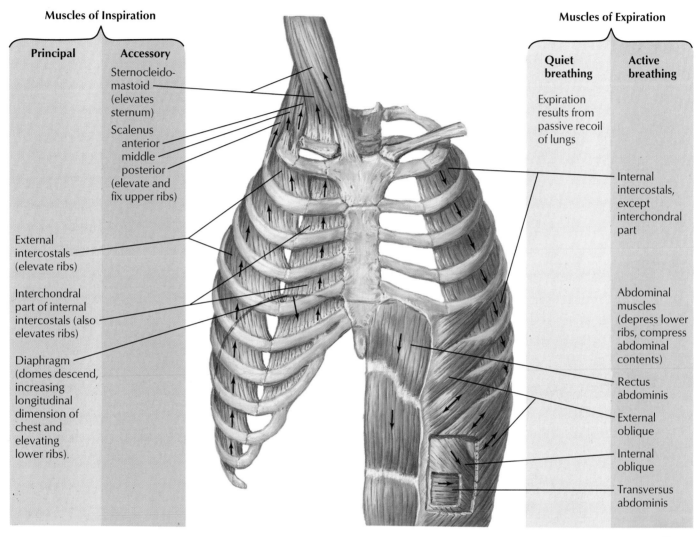

Muscles of Inspiration

Principal	Accessory
	Sternocleido-mastoid (elevates sternum)
	Scalenus anterior middle posterior (elevate and fix upper ribs)
External intercostals (elevate ribs)	
Interchondral part of internal intercostals (also elevates ribs)	
Diaphragm (domes descend, increasing longitudinal dimension of chest and elevating lower ribs).	

Muscles of Expiration

Quiet breathing	Active breathing
Expiration results from passive recoil of lungs	Internal intercostals, except interchondral part
	Abdominal muscles (depress lower ribs, compress abdominal contents)
	Rectus abdominis
	External oblique
	Internal oblique
	Transversus abdominis

FIGURE 5.5   RESPIRATORY MUSCLES

During quiet respiration, contraction of the diaphragm alone accounts for about 75% of inspiration. Muscles of the thoracic wall (intercostal muscles) and selected muscles of the neck and abdomen also can participate in inspiration and assist the diaphragm, especially during active breathing (e.g., during exercise).

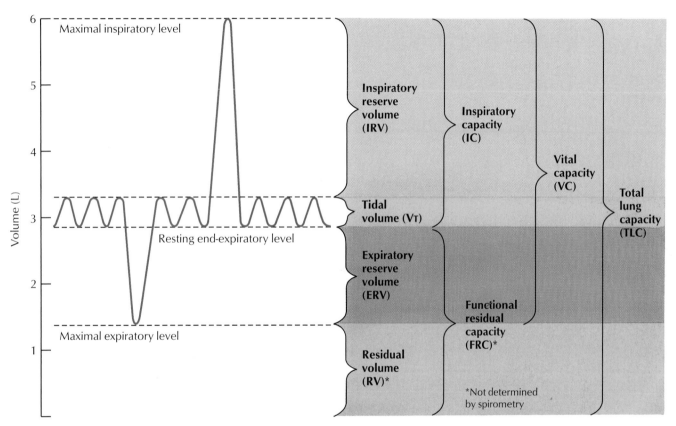

FIGURE 5.6   SPIROMETRY

Lung volumes are determined by spirometry. Shown are a number of normal tidal breaths, as well as one maximal inspiratory and one maximal expiratory breath. Typical volumes for an adult are shown.

A. At rest

1. Respiratory muscles are at rest
2. Recoil of lung and chest wall are equal but opposite
3. Pressure along tracheobronchial tree is atmospheric
4. There is no airflow

B. During inspiration

Inspiratory muscles contract and chest expands; alveolar pressure becomes subatmospheric with respect to pressure at airway opening. Air flows into lungs

C. During expiration

Inspiratory muscles relax; recoil of lung causes alveolar pressure to exceed pressure at airway opening. Air flows out of lung

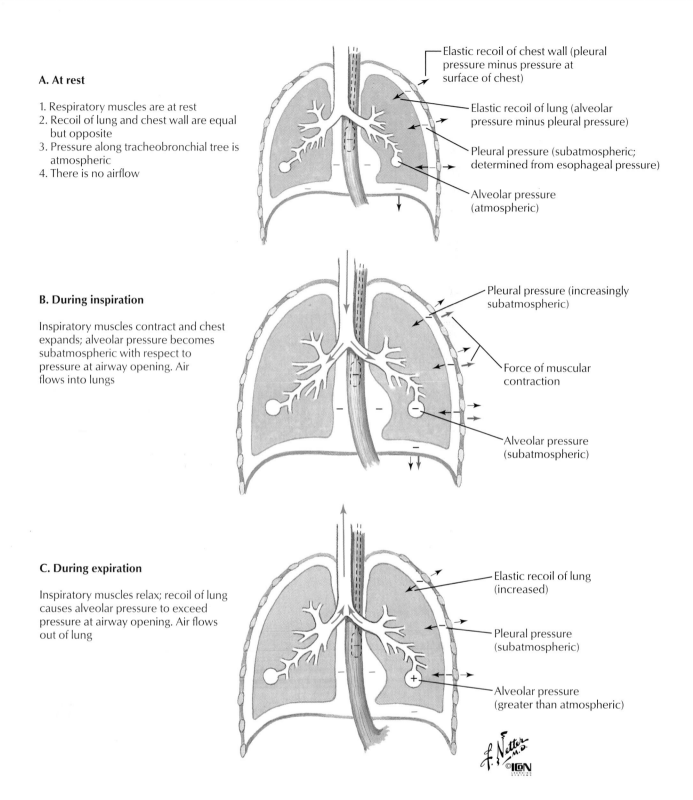

Elastic recoil of chest wall (pleural pressure minus pressure at surface of chest)

Elastic recoil of lung (alveolar pressure minus pleural pressure)

Pleural pressure (subatmospheric; determined from esophageal pressure)

Alveolar pressure (atmospheric)

Pleural pressure (increasingly subatmospheric)

Force of muscular contraction

Alveolar pressure (subatmospheric)

Elastic recoil of lung (increased)

Pleural pressure (subatmospheric)

Alveolar pressure (greater than atmospheric)

FIGURE 5.7 FORCES DURING QUIET BREATHING

The mechanics of ventilation involve the dynamic interaction of the lungs, chest wall, and diaphragm. The interplay of these structures and the resulting changes in pleural and alveolar pressures are depicted at rest and during inspiration and expiration.

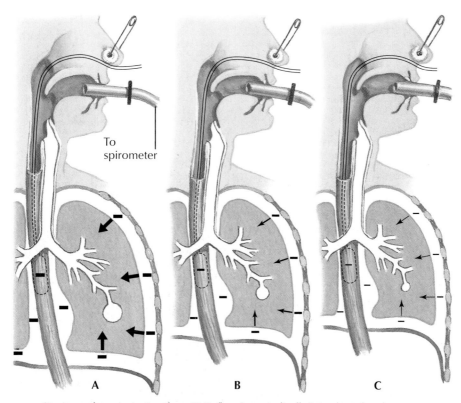

During a slow expiration from TLC, flow is periodically interrupted and measurements are made of lung volume and of transpulmonary pressure. Transpulmonary pressure is difference between alveolar and pleural pressures. Pleural pressure is determined from pressure in esophagus. Because there is no airflow, alveolar pressure is same as pressure at airway opening

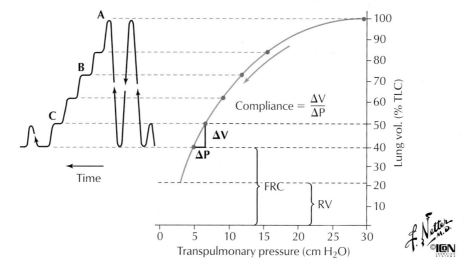

FIGURE 5.8 MEASUREMENT OF ELASTIC PROPERTIES OF LUNG

Compliance is a measure of the elasticity or distensibility of the lung, the chest wall, or the lung and chest wall as a single unit. It is measured as the change in volume resulting from a change in pressure ($\Delta V/\Delta P$). Depicted here is the measurement of the compli-ance of the lung. To measure lung compliance the change in lung volume is measured as the transpulmonary pressure (alveolar pres-sure − pleural pressure) varies during expiration. Pleural pressure is measured by a balloon placed in the esophagus.

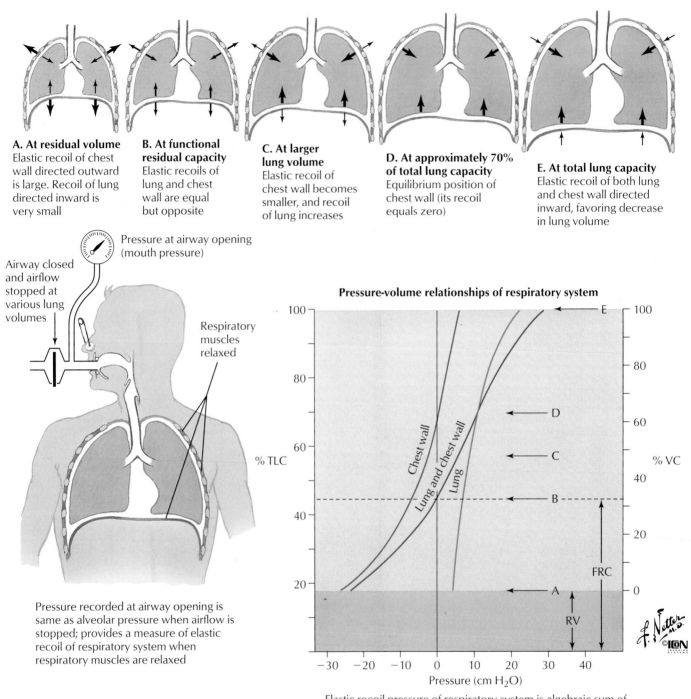

A. At residual volume
Elastic recoil of chest wall directed outward is large. Recoil of lung directed inward is very small

B. At functional residual capacity
Elastic recoils of lung and chest wall are equal but opposite

C. At larger lung volume
Elastic recoil of chest wall becomes smaller, and recoil of lung increases

D. At approximately 70% of total lung capacity
Equilibrium position of chest wall (its recoil equals zero)

E. At total lung capacity
Elastic recoil of both lung and chest wall directed inward, favoring decrease in lung volume

Pressure at airway opening (mouth pressure)

Airway closed and airflow stopped at various lung volumes

Respiratory muscles relaxed

Pressure recorded at airway opening is same as alveolar pressure when airflow is stopped; provides a measure of elastic recoil of respiratory system when respiratory muscles are relaxed

Pressure-volume relationships of respiratory system

% TLC

% VC

Chest wall

Lung and chest wall

Lung

FRC

RV

Pressure (cm H_2O)

Elastic recoil pressure of respiratory system is algebraic sum of recoil pressures of lung and chest wall

FIGURE 5.9   ELASTIC PROPERTIES OF RESPIRATORY SYSTEM: LUNG AND CHEST WALL

The elastic recoil (or compliance) properties of the lungs and chest wall alone and combined are shown diagrammatically and graphically.

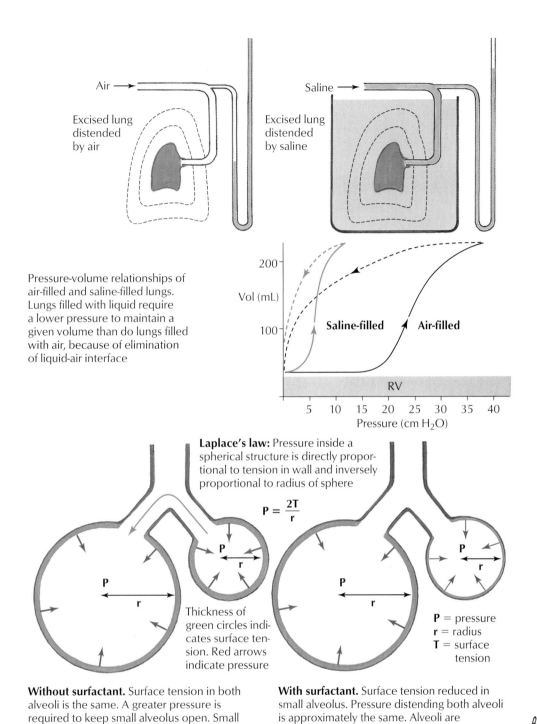

Pressure-volume relationships of air-filled and saline-filled lungs. Lungs filled with liquid require a lower pressure to maintain a given volume than do lungs filled with air, because of elimination of liquid-air interface

Laplace's law: Pressure inside a spherical structure is directly proportional to tension in wall and inversely proportional to radius of sphere

$$P = \frac{2T}{r}$$

Thickness of green circles indicates surface tension. Red arrows indicate pressure

P = pressure
r = radius
T = surface tension

Without surfactant. Surface tension in both alveoli is the same. A greater pressure is required to keep small alveolus open. Small alveolus tends to empty into larger one

With surfactant. Surface tension reduced in small alveolus. Pressure distending both alveoli is approximately the same. Alveoli are stabilized, and the tendency for small alveolus to empty into larger one is reduced

FIGURE 5.10   SURFACE FORCES IN THE LUNG

The alveoli are coated with a thin film of surfactant (lipoprotein produced by type 2 alveolar cells). Surfactant reduces the surface tension that exists at the air-alveolar interface. This has several effects, including a decrease in elastic recoil of the lung, an increase in lung compliance, and a decrease in the work required to inflate the lung during inspiration. Surfactants' effect on surface tension is greater in small alveoli compared with large alveoli. This tends to stabilize the alveoli and thereby equalize alveolar pressures throughout the lung.

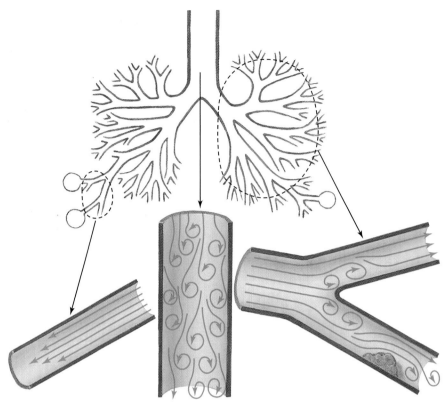

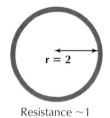

Laminar flow occurs mainly in small peripheral airways where rate of airflow through any airway is low. Driving pressure is proportional to gas viscosity

Turbulent flow occurs at high flow rates in trachea and larger airways. Driving pressure is proportional to square of flow and is dependent on gas density

Transitional flow occurs in larger airways, particularly at branches and at sites of narrowing. Driving pressure is proportional to both gas density and gas viscosity

Poiseuille's law. Resistance to laminar flow is inversely proportional to tube radius to the 4th power and directly proportional to length of tube. When radius is halved, resistance is increased 16-fold. If driving pressure is constant, flow will fall to one sixteenth. Doubling length only doubles resistance. If driving pressure is constant, flow will fall to one half

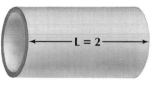

Resistance ~1

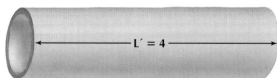

Resistance ~16

Resistance ~2

Resistance ~4

FIGURE 5.11   AIRWAY FLOW

Airflow through the large airways of the lung is turbulent and therefore can be heard with a stethoscope (i.e., breath sounds). Laminar flow occurs only in the small airways. The major factor that determines resistance to airflow is the diameter of the airway, because resistance varies as the fourth power of the radius.

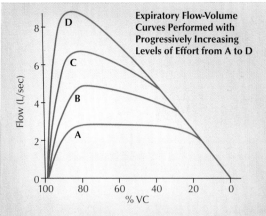

Expiratory Flow-Volume Curves Performed with Progressively Increasing Levels of Effort from A to D

At high lung volumes, rate of airflow during expiration increases progressively with increasing effort. At intermediate and low lung volumes, airflow reaches maximal levels after only modest effort is exerted and thereafter increases no further despite increasing effort

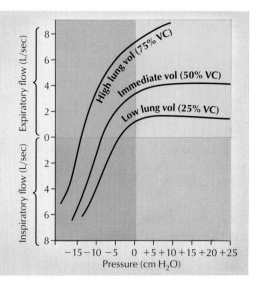

Isovolume Pressure-Flow Curves

At lung volumes greater than 75% of VC, airflow increases progressively with increasing pleural pressure. Airflow is effort dependent. At volumes below 75% of VC, airflow levels off as pleural pressure exceeds atmospheric pressure. Thereafter, airflow is effort independent, because further increases in pleural pressure result in no further rise in rate of airflow

Determinants of Maximal Expiratory Flow

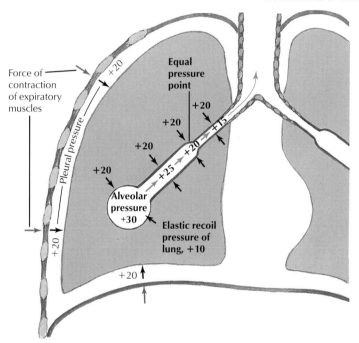

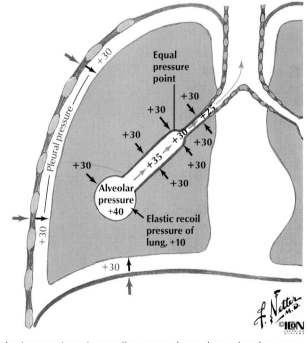

At onset of maximal airflow contraction of expiratory muscles at a given lung volume raises pleural pressure above atmospheric level (+20 cm H₂O). Alveolar pressure (sum of pleural pressure and lung recoil pressure) is yet higher (+30 cm H₂O). Airway pressure falls progressively from alveolus to airway opening in overcoming resistance. At equal pressure point of airway, pressure within airway equals pressure surrounding it (pleural pressure). Beyond this point, as intraluminal pressure drops further, below pleural pressure, airway will be compressed

With further increases in expiratory effort, at same lung volume, pleural pressure is greater and alveolar pressure is correspondingly higher. Fall in airway pressure and location of equal pressure point are unchanged, but beyond equal pressure point, intrathoracic airways will be compressed to a greater degree by higher pleural pressure. Once maximal airflow is achieved, further increases in pleural pressure produce proportional increases in resistance of segment downstream from equal pressure point, so rate of airflow does not change

---

FIGURE 5.12   FLOW-VOLUME RELATIONSHIPS

Airflow varies as a function of pressure and lung volume. The highest rates of airflow are seen at high lung volumes.

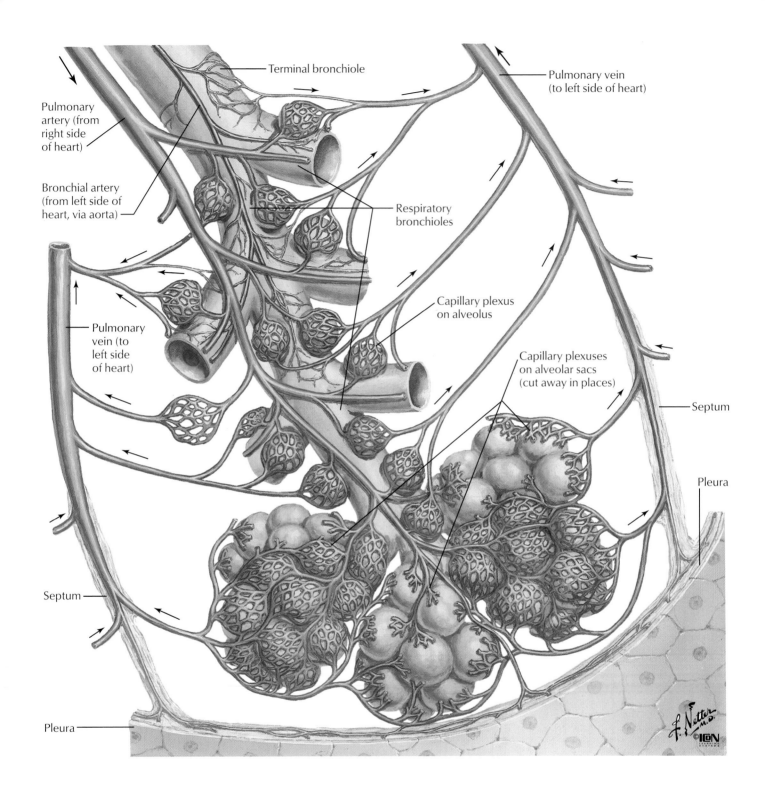

FIGURE 5.13   INTRAPULMONARY BLOOD CIRCULATION

Blood from the right ventricle of the heart perfuses the lungs (via the pulmonary artery) at a relatively high rate (approximately 5 L/min) but under low pressure (driving pressure of about 6 mm Hg). Pulmonary capillary plexuses envelop the alveolar sacs, where most of the gas exchange occurs. Pulmonary veins collect the oxygenated blood and return it to the left side of the heart for distribution to the systemic circulation. In a normal resting adult, the lungs contain about 75 mL of blood distributed variably across its vasculature.

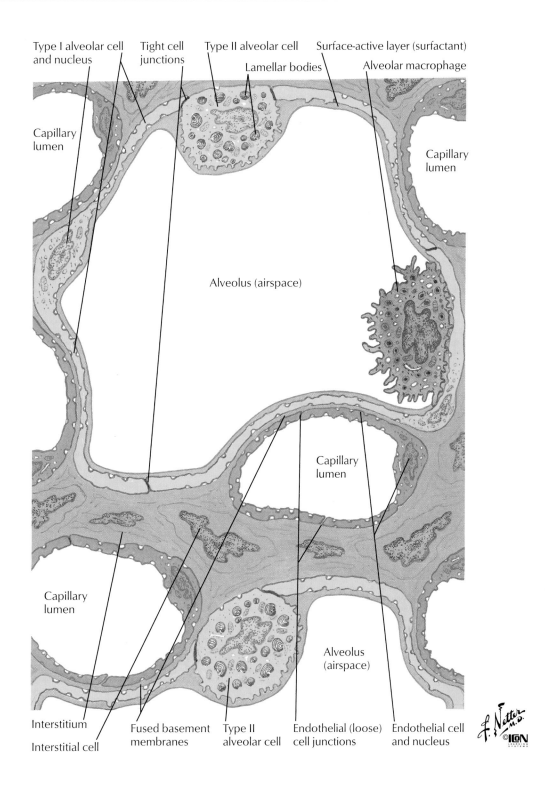

FIGURE 5.14   ULTRASTRUCTURE OF PULMONARY ALVEOLI AND CAPILLARIES

Gas exchange occurs across the type I alveolar cells, the basement membrane, and the capillary endothelial cell. The type II alveolar cells secrete surfactant, which forms a thin layer over the fluid that coats the surface of the alveolus. Alveolar macrophages migrate out of the capillaries and can be found in the interstitium of the alveolar septa or within the alveolus itself. They serve to engulf inhaled particulates and bacteria.

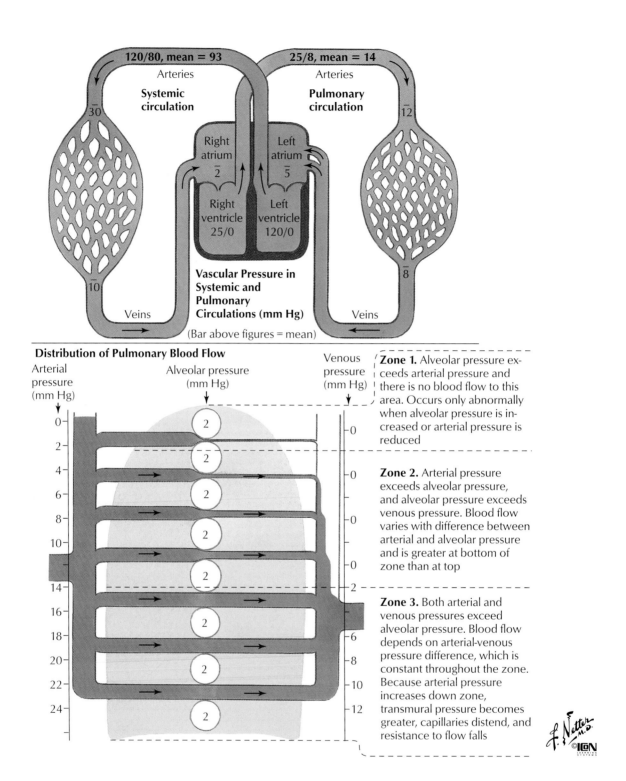

Vascular Pressure in Systemic and Pulmonary Circulations (mm Hg)

(Bar above figures = mean)

Distribution of Pulmonary Blood Flow

Zone 1. Alveolar pressure exceeds arterial pressure and there is no blood flow to this area. Occurs only abnormally when alveolar pressure is increased or arterial pressure is reduced

Zone 2. Arterial pressure exceeds alveolar pressure, and alveolar pressure exceeds venous pressure. Blood flow varies with difference between arterial and alveolar pressure and is greater at bottom of zone than at top

Zone 3. Both arterial and venous pressures exceed alveolar pressure. Blood flow depends on arterial-venous pressure difference, which is constant throughout the zone. Because arterial pressure increases down zone, transmural pressure becomes greater, capillaries distend, and resistance to flow falls

FIGURE 5.15   PULMONARY CIRCULATION

Due to the effects of gravity, blood flow is not evenly distributed throughout the lung. As a result, the capillaries in the apex of the lung are not perfused, and those at the base are distended.

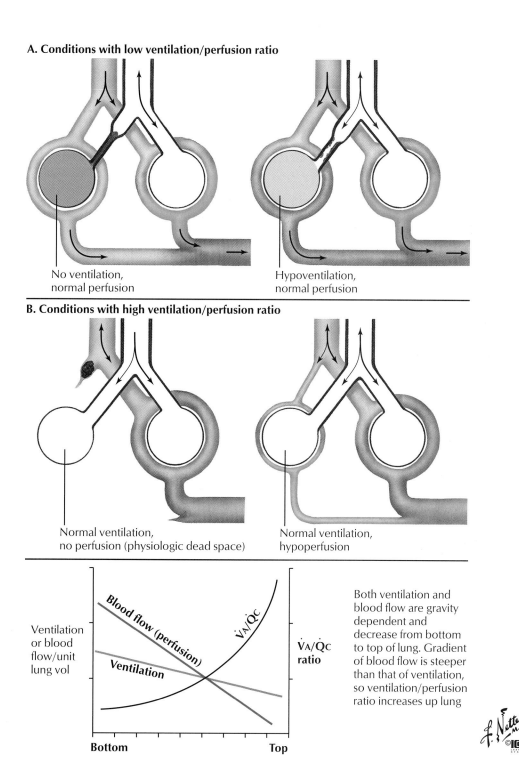

A. Conditions with low ventilation/perfusion ratio

No ventilation,
normal perfusion

Hypoventilation,
normal perfusion

B. Conditions with high ventilation/perfusion ratio

Normal ventilation,
no perfusion (physiologic dead space)

Normal ventilation,
hypoperfusion

Ventilation
or blood
flow/unit
lung vol

Blood flow (perfusion)

$\dot{V}A/\dot{Q}C$

Ventilation

$\dot{V}A/\dot{Q}C$
ratio

Bottom

Top

Both ventilation and
blood flow are gravity
dependent and
decrease from bottom
to top of lung. Gradient
of blood flow is steeper
than that of ventilation,
so ventilation/perfusion
ratio increases up lung

FIGURE 5.16   VENTILATION/PERFUSION ($\dot{V}a/\dot{Q}c$) RELATIONSHIPS

Gravity affects not only capillary perfusion (see Figure 5.15) but alveolar ventilation as well. In an erect person the ratio of ventilation to perfusion ($\dot{V}a/\dot{Q}c$) is greater than 1 at the apices (i.e., high ventilation but low blood flow), whereas the opposite is true at the bases. In a normal lung the average $\dot{V}a/\dot{Q}c$ is approximately 1.

Effects of chemical and humoral substances

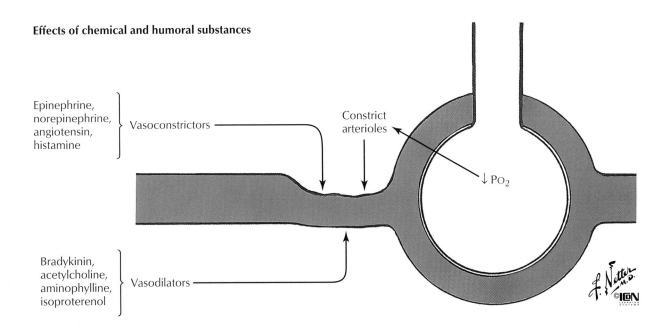

Epinephrine, norepinephrine, angiotensin, histamine — Vasoconstrictors

Bradykinin, acetylcholine, aminophylline, isoproterenol — Vasodilators

Constrict arterioles

$\downarrow PO_2$

FIGURE 5.17   PULMONARY VASCULAR RESISTANCE

Pulmonary vascular resistance is influenced by a number of substances. Importantly, a decrease in alveolar PO_2 constricts the arterioles perfusing that alveolus. This is in contrast to all other vascular beds in the body, where a decrease on PO_2 dilates arterioles. This unique response of the pulmonary arterioles to a decrease in alveolar PO_2 helps ensure that the capillaries of nonaerated alveoli are not perfused.

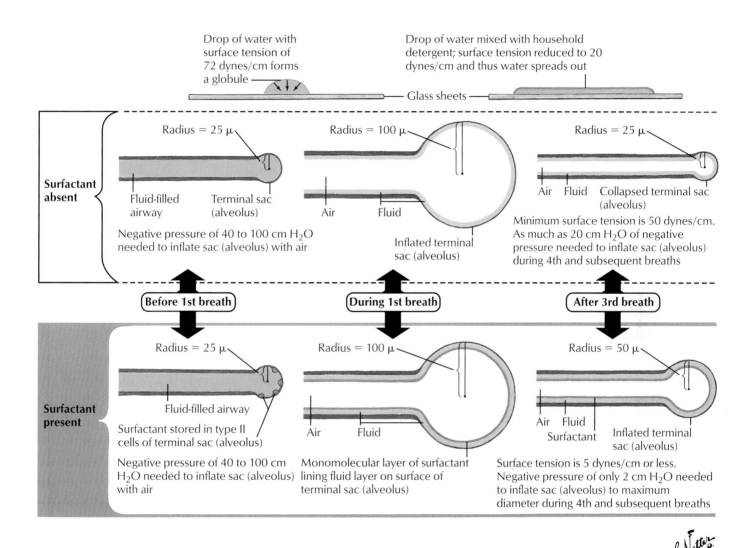

Drop of water with surface tension of 72 dynes/cm forms a globule

Drop of water mixed with household detergent; surface tension reduced to 20 dynes/cm and thus water spreads out

Glass sheets

Surfactant absent

Radius = 25 μ

Fluid-filled airway

Terminal sac (alveolus)

Negative pressure of 40 to 100 cm H₂O needed to inflate sac (alveolus) with air

Radius = 100 μ

Air   Fluid

Inflated terminal sac (alveolus)

Radius = 25 μ

Air   Fluid   Collapsed terminal sac (alveolus)

Minimum surface tension is 50 dynes/cm. As much as 20 cm H₂O of negative pressure needed to inflate sac (alveolus) during 4th and subsequent breaths

Before 1st breath   **During 1st breath**   **After 3rd breath**

Surfactant present

Radius = 25 μ

Fluid-filled airway

Surfactant stored in type II cells of terminal sac (alveolus)

Negative pressure of 40 to 100 cm H₂O needed to inflate sac (alveolus) with air

Radius = 100 μ

Air   Fluid

Monomolecular layer of surfactant lining fluid layer on surface of terminal sac (alveolus)

Radius = 50 μ

Air   Fluid
Surfactant   Inflated terminal sac (alveolus)

Surface tension is 5 dynes/cm or less. Negative pressure of only 2 cm H₂O needed to inflate sac (alveolus) to maximum diameter during 4th and subsequent breaths

FIGURE 5.18   SURFACTANT EFFECTS

Surfactant is produced by type II alveolar cells (see Figure 5.14). Its major component is the phospholipid dipalmitoyl phosphatidylcholine. It acts to reduce the surface tension of the fluid-lined alveoli (see also Figure 5.10). Thus, lower pressures are required to inflate the alveoli. Failure to produce sufficient amounts of surfactant, as can occur in premature infants, results in an increase in the work of breathing and respiratory distress.

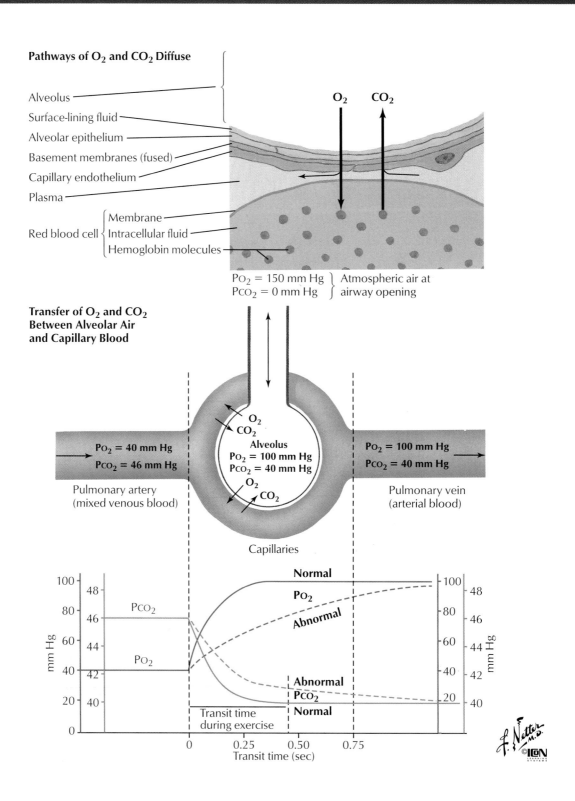

Pathways of O₂ and CO₂ Diffuse

Alveolus
Surface-lining fluid
Alveolar epithelium
Basement membranes (fused)
Capillary endothelium
Plasma
Red blood cell {
Membrane
Intracellular fluid
Hemoglobin molecules

O₂   CO₂

P_{O_2} = 150 mm Hg ⎫ Atmospheric air at
P_{CO_2} = 0 mm Hg ⎭ airway opening

Transfer of O₂ and CO₂ Between Alveolar Air and Capillary Blood

P_{O_2} = 40 mm Hg
P_{CO_2} = 46 mm Hg

Pulmonary artery
(mixed venous blood)

O₂
CO₂
Alveolus
P_{O_2} = 100 mm Hg
P_{CO_2} = 40 mm Hg
O₂
CO₂

P_{O_2} = 100 mm Hg
P_{CO_2} = 40 mm Hg

Pulmonary vein
(arterial blood)

Capillaries

Normal
Po₂
Abnormal

mm Hg

P_{CO_2}

P_{O_2}

Abnormal
Pco₂
Normal

Transit time
during exercise

0   0.25   0.50   0.75
Transit time (sec)

FIGURE 5.19   O₂ AND CO₂ EXCHANGE

As blood flows through the alveolar capillary, O₂ diffuses from the alveolus into the red blood cell, where it binds to hemoglobin. At the same time, CO₂ diffuses out of the red blood cell and into the alveolus. Normally, blood traverses the entire length of the capillary in 0.75 second. With increased cardiac output, the transit time is reduced. Full equilibration of blood with alveolar O₂ and CO₂ still occurs with transit times as low as 0.5 second. In some disease states there is thickening of the alveolar-capillary wall. This restricts the diffusion of O₂ and CO₂ and can prevent full equilibration of blood with the alveolar gases during the time required for the blood to travel the length of the capillary (dashed lines labeled as abnormal).

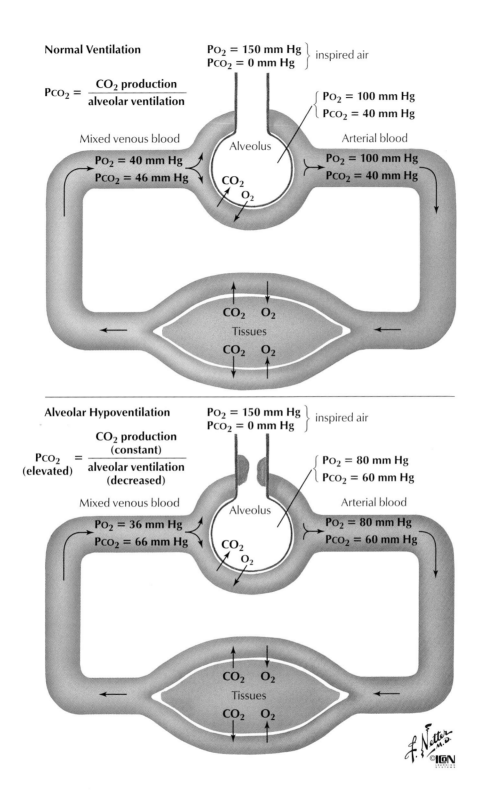

Normal Ventilation

$$P_{CO_2} = \frac{CO_2 \text{ production}}{\text{alveolar ventilation}}$$

$P_{O_2} = 150$ mm Hg
$P_{CO_2} = 0$ mm Hg $\Big\}$ inspired air

$P_{O_2} = 100$ mm Hg
$P_{CO_2} = 40$ mm Hg

Mixed venous blood

$P_{O_2} = 40$ mm Hg
$P_{CO_2} = 46$ mm Hg

Alveolus

Arterial blood

$P_{O_2} = 100$ mm Hg
$P_{CO_2} = 40$ mm Hg

CO_2
O_2

$CO_2 \quad O_2$
Tissues
$CO_2 \quad O_2$

Alveolar Hypoventilation

$$P_{CO_2} \atop \text{(elevated)} = \frac{CO_2 \text{ production (constant)}}{\text{alveolar ventilation (decreased)}}$$

$P_{O_2} = 150$ mm Hg
$P_{CO_2} = 0$ mm Hg $\Big\}$ inspired air

$P_{O_2} = 80$ mm Hg
$P_{CO_2} = 60$ mm Hg

Mixed venous blood

$P_{O_2} = 36$ mm Hg
$P_{CO_2} = 66$ mm Hg

Alveolus

Arterial blood

$P_{O_2} = 80$ mm Hg
$P_{CO_2} = 60$ mm Hg

CO_2
O_2

$CO_2 \quad O_2$
Tissues
$CO_2 \quad O_2$

F. Netter
M.D.
©ICON
LEARNING
SYSTEMS

FIGURE 5.20   O₂ AND CO₂ EXCHANGE AND TRANSPORT

Alveolar hypoventilation, illustrated here as a partial blockage of the airway, reduces the alveolar P_{O_2} and increases the alveolar P_{CO_2}. As a result, the arterial blood P_{O_2} declines (hypoxia) and the arterial blood P_{CO_2} increases (hypercapnia).

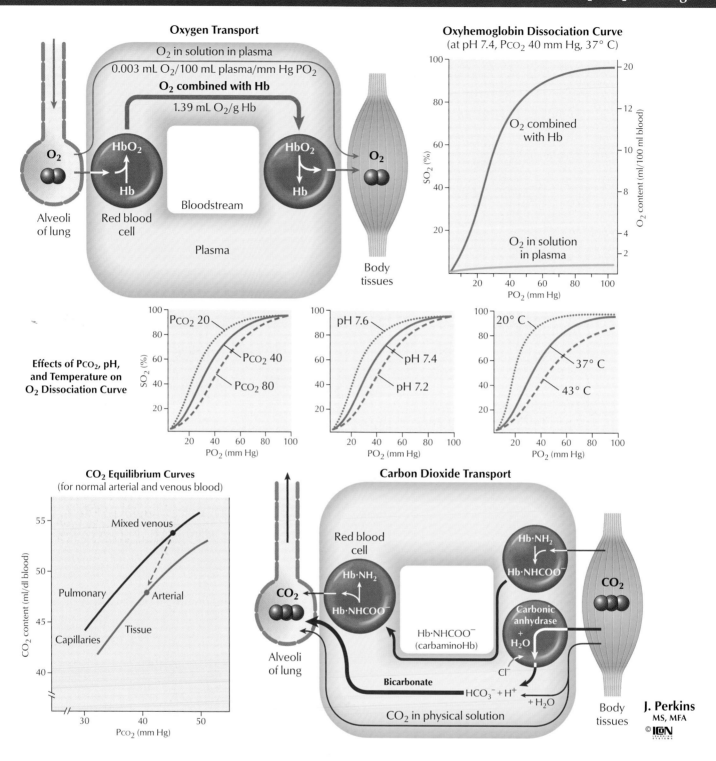

FIGURE 5.21 O₂/CO₂ EXCHANGE

During each breath, O_2 and CO_2 are exchanged across the alveolar-pulmonary capillary membrane (see Figure 5.19). Almost all of the O_2 carried to the tissues is bound to hemoglobin (Hb); only a small amount is dissolved and transported in plasma. As shown in the oxyhemoglobin dissociation curve, the binding of O_2 to Hb is dependent on the partial pressure of O_2 (P_{O_2}). The percent saturation of Hb (S_{O_2}) is about 97.5% when the P_{O_2} is 100 mm Hg. In the three middle panels, the effects of CO_2, pH, and temperature on the oxyhemoglobin dissociation curve are shown. Hb binding of

O_2 is decreased, and thereby off-loading of O_2 to the tissues is increased by increased P_{CO_2} (hypercapnia), decreased pH (acidosis), or increased body temperature (fever). CO_2 from the tissues is transported largely in the form of HCO_3^-. A small amount is transported in the dissolved form, and some is carried in the form of carbaminohemoglobin. The bottom left panel shows that the CO_2 equilibrium (dissociation) curve is much steeper than that for O_2, which is why the P_{CO_2} difference between arterial and mixed venous blood is small (about 5 mm Hg).

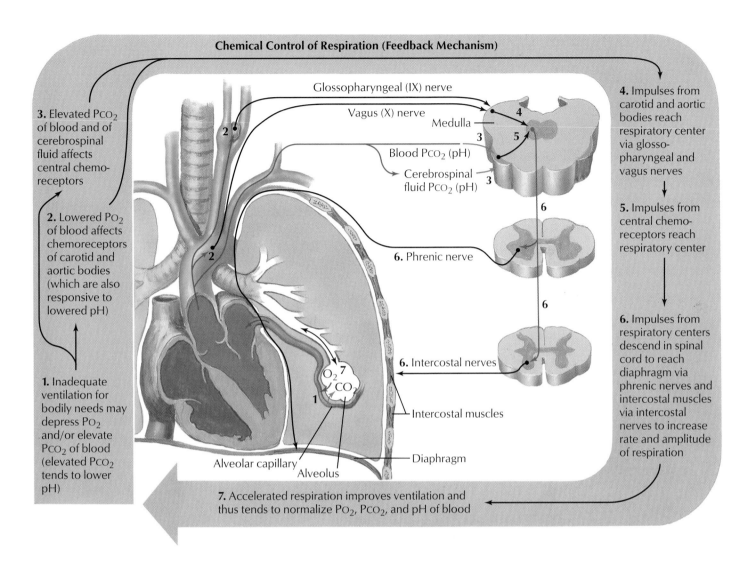

Chemical Control of Respiration (Feedback Mechanism)

Glossopharyngeal (IX) nerve

Vagus (X) nerve

Medulla

Blood P_{CO_2} (pH)

Cerebrospinal fluid P_{CO_2} (pH)

3. Elevated P_{CO_2} of blood and of cerebrospinal fluid affects central chemoreceptors

2. Lowered P_{O_2} of blood affects chemoreceptors of carotid and aortic bodies (which are also responsive to lowered pH)

1. Inadequate ventilation for bodily needs may depress P_{O_2} and/or elevate P_{CO_2} of blood (elevated P_{CO_2} tends to lower pH)

6. Phrenic nerve

O_2 CO_2

6. Intercostal nerves

Intercostal muscles

Alveolar capillary

Alveolus

Diaphragm

4. Impulses from carotid and aortic bodies reach respiratory center via glossopharyngeal and vagus nerves

5. Impulses from central chemoreceptors reach respiratory center

6. Impulses from respiratory centers descend in spinal cord to reach diaphragm via phrenic nerves and intercostal muscles via intercostal nerves to increase rate and amplitude of respiration

7. Accelerated respiration improves ventilation and thus tends to normalize P_{O_2}, P_{CO_2}, and pH of blood

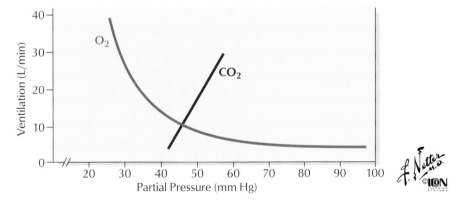

FIGURE 5.22   CONTROL OF RESPIRATION

The central chemoreceptors respond to changes in arterial P_{CO_2}, but not arterial P_{O_2} or pH. Elevated P_{CO_2} of arterial blood stimulates central brainstem chemoreceptors via changes in the pH of the cerebrospinal and brain interstitial fluid. The increased P_{CO_2} results in a decrease in pH, and this in turn increases the rate and amplitude of respiration. Peripheral chemoreceptors (carotid and aortic bodies) sense changes in the arterial blood P_{CO_2}, P_{O_2}, and pH, and send signals via the glossopharyngeal and vagus nerves to the brainstem respiratory centers. The increase in respiratory rate and amplitude seen with a decrease in arterial P_{O_2} (hypoxia) or a decrease in arterial pH is mediated by the peripheral chemoreceptors.

111

A. Role of Lungs and Kidneys in Acid-Base Balance

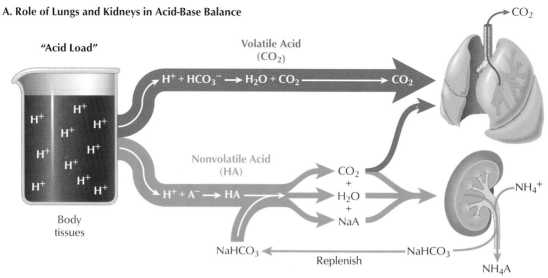

"Acid Load"

Volatile Acid (CO_2)

CO_2

$$H^+ + HCO_3^- \rightarrow H_2O + CO_2 \rightarrow CO_2$$

Body tissues

Nonvolatile Acid (HA)

$$H^+ + A^- \rightarrow HA$$

CO_2 + H_2O + NaA

NH_4^+

$NaHCO_3 \leftarrow$ Replenish $\leftarrow NaHCO_3$

NH_4A

B. Metabolic Production of Acid and Alkali

Food Source	Acid/Alkali	Quantity (mEq/day)
Carbohydrate ⎤ Fat ⎦ → CO_2		15 - 20,000
Amino acids		
S-containing	H_2SO_4 ⎤	
Cationic	HCl ⎬ →	100 (acid)
Anionic	HCO_3^- ⎦	
Organic ions	HCO_3^-	60 (alkali)
Phosphate	$H_2PO_4^-$	30 (acid)
Total		**70 (acid)**

1 mEq/kg/day of nonvolatile acid production

C. Acid-Base Paths

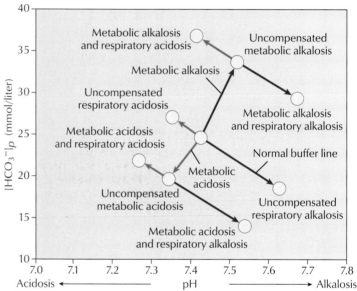

$[HCO_3^-]_p$ (mmol/liter)

Metabolic alkalosis and respiratory acidosis

Uncompensated metabolic alkalosis

Metabolic alkalosis

Uncompensated respiratory acidosis

Metabolic alkalosis and respiratory alkalosis

Metabolic acidosis and respiratory acidosis

Normal buffer line

Metabolic acidosis

Uncompensated metabolic acidosis

Uncompensated respiratory alkalosis

Metabolic acidosis and respiratory alkalosis

Acidosis ←   pH   → Alkalosis

D. Acid-Base Disorders

Disorder	pH	1° Alteration	Defense Mechanisms
Metabolic acidosis	↓	↓ [HCO_3^-]	Buffers, ↓ PCO_2, ↑NAE
Metabolic alkalosis	↑	↑ [HCO_3^-]	Buffers, ↑ PCO_2, ↓NAE
Respiratory acidosis	↓	↑ PCO_2	Buffers & ↑NAE
Respiratory alkalosis	↑	↓ PCO_2	Buffers & ↓NAE

J. Perkins
MS, MFA
©ICN

FIGURE 5.23   ACID-BASE BALANCE

A, Both the lungs and kidneys participate in acid-base balance. *B,* Our diet and cellular metabolism add acid and alkali to our system. In a typical meat-containing diet, there is the addition of acid to our body fluids. CO_2 (sometimes referred to as "volatile acid"), generated by carbohydrate and fat metabolism, is efficiently eliminated by the lungs and does not normally affect acid-base balance. However, failure to excrete the CO_2 can alter acid-base balance. Nonvolatile acid (e.g., lactic acid) is buffered by HCO_3^- in the extracellular fluid. The kidneys must excrete this nonvolatile acid and replenish the HCO_3^- used to neutralize these acids. The kidneys do this by excreting the acid anion with NH_4^+ (the kidneys also excrete H^+, which also results in the addition HCO_3^- to the extracellular fluid (see Figure 6.18). The lungs serve as a respiratory "buffer" that can respond quickly and remove large quantities of volatile acid (CO_2) by hyperventilation. The kidneys take hours or days to respond to an acid-base imbalance and do so largely by varying the amount of NH_4^+ excreted in the urine. *C* and *D* illustrate acid-base disorders resulting from alterations in the PCO_2 (respiratory disorders) or alterations in the [HCO_3^-] (metabolic disorders). When an acid-base disturbance occurs, intracellular (primarily proteins) and extracellular (primarily HCO_3^-) buffers minimize the change in body fluid pH. In addition, the lungs can adjust the PCO_2 to compensate for metabolic disorders, and the kidneys can adjust net acid excretion to compensate for respiratory disorders. *Note:* Net acid excretion (NAE) includes acid excreted with urinary buffers and as NH_4^+, less any HCO_3^- lost in the urine.

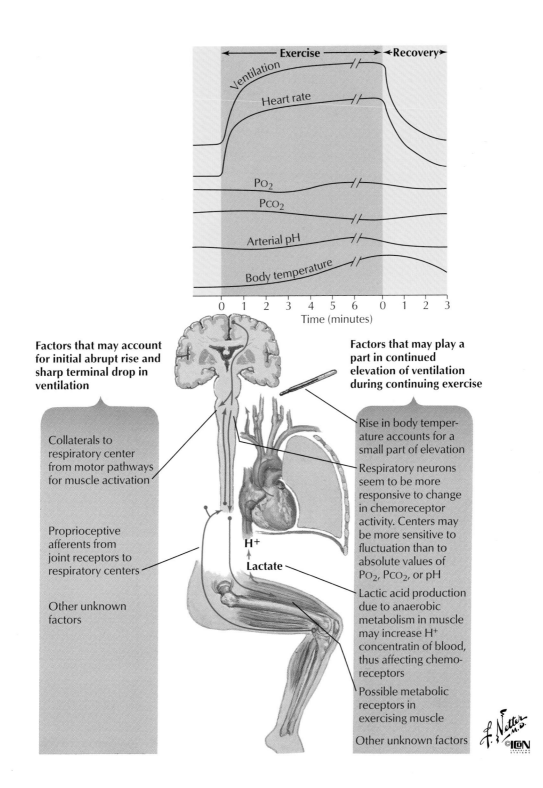

Factors that may account for initial abrupt rise and sharp terminal drop in ventilation

Collaterals to respiratory center from motor pathways for muscle activation

Proprioceptive afferents from joint receptors to respiratory centers

Other unknown factors

Factors that may play a part in continued elevation of ventilation during continuing exercise

Rise in body temperature accounts for a small part of elevation

Respiratory neurons seem to be more responsive to change in chemoreceptor activity. Centers may be more sensitive to fluctuation than to absolute values of P_{O_2}, P_{CO_2}, or pH

Lactic acid production due to anaerobic metabolism in muscle may increase H^+ concentratin of blood, thus affecting chemo-receptors

Possible metabolic receptors in exercising muscle

Other unknown factors

H^+

↑
Lactate

FIGURE 5.24   RESPIRATORY RESPONSE TO EXERCISE

Exercise increases the demand for delivery of O_2 to the tissues and the excretion of CO_2, both of which require an increase in the ventilatory rate. The ventilatory rate increases concurrently with the exercise-induced increase in cardiac output (represented here as an increase in heart rate). A number of factors are involved in this response and are indicated.

Centriacinar (Centrilobular) Emphysema

Magnified section. Distended, inter-communicating, saclike spaces in central area of acini

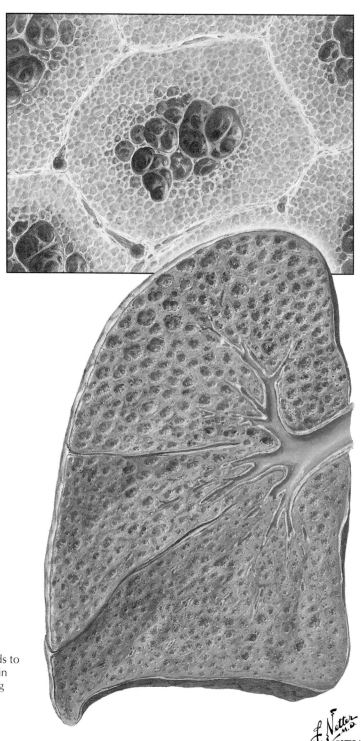

Gross specimen. Involvement tends to be most marked in upper part of lung

FIGURE 5.25　OBSTRUCTIVE DISEASE: EMPHYSEMA

This figure shows the gross and microscopic appearance of a lung as it appears in a person with centriacinar (centrolobular) emphysema. Note the dilated air spaces and rupture of the alveolar walls.

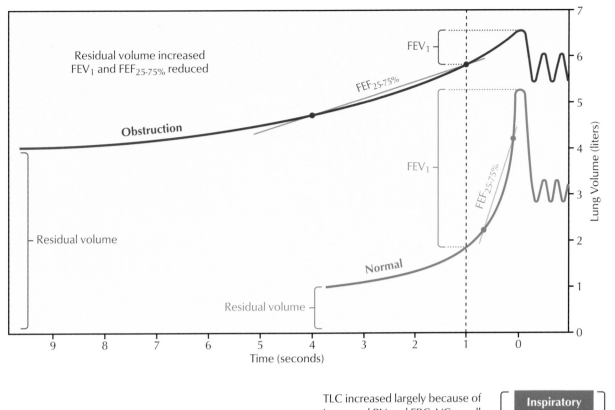

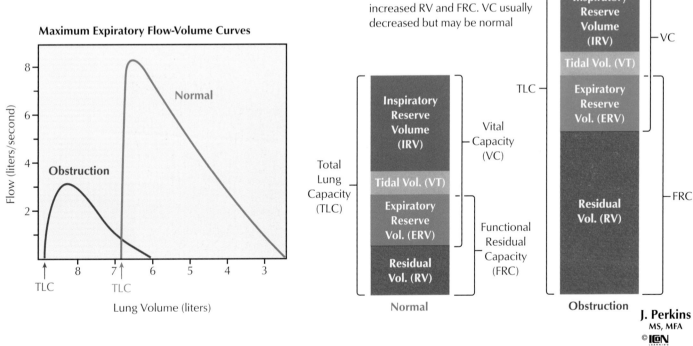

J. Perkins
MS, MFA
©ICON

FIGURE 5.26 OBSTRUCTIVE LUNG DISEASE

Obstructive pulmonary disease refers to a group of conditions (e.g., emphysema, chronic bronchitis, and asthma), all of which cause shortness of breath and obstruction of airflow. Shown here is the effect of severe emphysema on pulmonary function. In emphysema, inflammatory processes destroy the connective tissue of the lung, and in particular the elastic fibers that help maintain the patency of the airways (i.e., elastic recoil). Therefore, lung compliance is increased. The decreased elastic recoil results in collapse of airways during expiration (a process termed dynamic compression; see Figure 5.12) and air trapping. The trapped air results in an increase in TLC and FRC as a result of a large increase in RV. In addition, dynamic compression of the airway prolongs the forced expiratory volume in the first second (FEV_1), as well as the force expiratory flow rate measured over the middle half of expiration ($FEF_{25-75\%}$). Because the VC (measured as forced vital capacity [FVC]) is only slightly decreased, or even normal, the ratio of FEV_1/FVC is typically less than 75%.

115

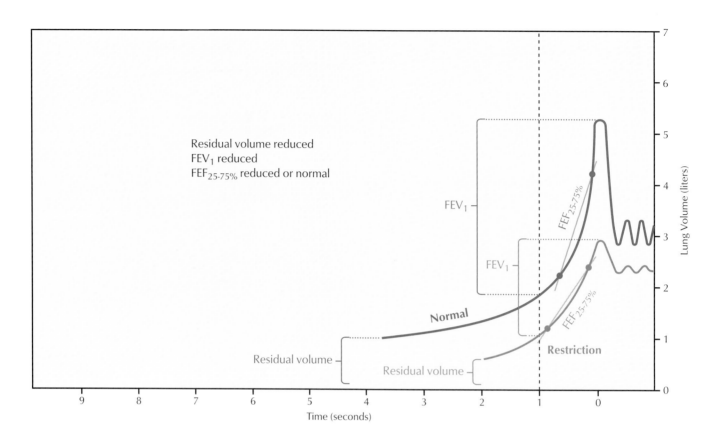

Residual volume reduced
FEV₁ reduced
FEF₂₅₋₇₅% reduced or normal

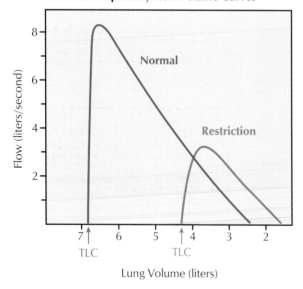

Maximum Expiratory Flow-Volume Curves

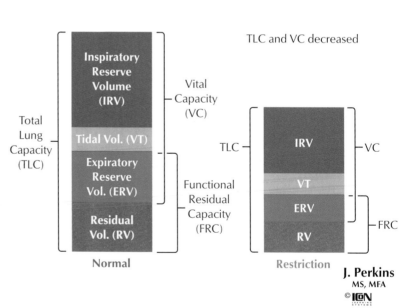

TLC and VC decreased

J. Perkins
MS, MFA
© ICN

FIGURE 5.27 RESTRICTIVE PULMONARY DISEASE

Restrictive pulmonary disease refers to a group of disorders that result in an increase in the connective tissue of the lung (e.g., fibrosis, alveolar wall thickening). The increased connective tissue reduces lung compliance, making it increasingly difficult to expand the lung during inspiration. As a result, virtually all lung volumes are reduced. In particular, as shown here, there can be marked decreases in TLC and VC (measured as forced vital capacity [FVC]). The forced expiratory volume in the first second (FEV₁) is decreased in proportion to FVC, so the ratio of FEV₁/FVC is typically normal. If the FVC is markedly decreased, this ratio may even increase.

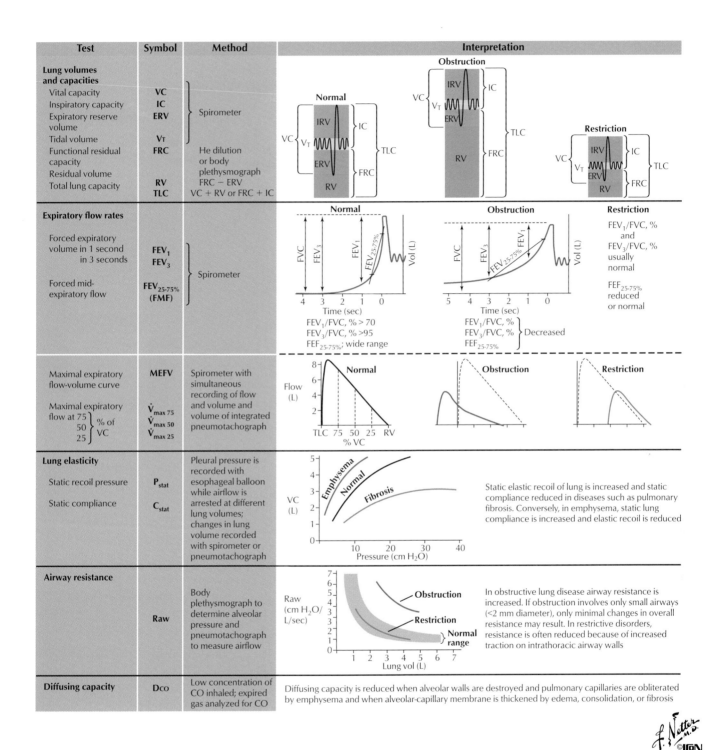

FIGURE 5.28 TESTS OF PULMONARY FUNCTION

This figure illustrates pulmonary function tests and comparative values for normal lungs and diseased lungs (obstructive or restrictive disease).

Test	Symbol	Method	Interpretation		
Tests for small airway disease Closing volume Closing capacity	**CV** **CC**	Following a full inspiration of O_2 the expired lung volume from TLC to RV is plotted against the N_2 concentration		Airways in the lower lung zones close at low lung volumes and only those alveoli at top of lungs continue to empty. Because concentration of N_2 in alveoli of upper zones is higher, the slope of the curve abruptly increases (phase IV). Phase IV begins at larger lung volumes in individuals with even minor degrees of airway obstruction increasing both CV and CC	
Maximal expiratory flow-volume curve breathing 80% He and 20% O_2	$\Delta\dot{V}_{max\ 50}$ V iso $\dot{V}$	Spirometer or pneumotachograph to record flow and volume	 During a maximal expiratory maneuver, resistance to airflow is normally due to turbulence and convective acceleration. Breathing He, which is less dense than air, lowers resistance and increases flow at all but the lowest volumes. In small airway disease, resistance to laminar flow makes up larger portion of total resistance and airflow is relatively independent of gas density. Increase in expiratory flow at 50% of VC while breathing He-O_2 ($\Delta\dot{V}_{max\ 50}$) will be less, and volume at which flows while breathing He-O_2 and while breathing air are identical (V iso $\dot{V}$) will be higher in patients with small airway disease than in normal individuals		

Test	Symbol	Method	Normal values	Abnormalities
Gas exchange Partial pressure of O_2 in arterial blood	Po_2	Arterial blood is collected anaerobically in heparinized syringe	60 to 100 mm Hg breathing room air at sea level; falls slightly with age	Hypoxemia indicative of ventilation/perfusion abnormalities, shunts, diffusion defect, alveolar hypoventilation
Partial pressure of CO_2 in arterial blood	Pco_2		36 to 44 mm Hg	Pco_2 proportional to metabolic rate (CO_2 production) and inversely related to volume of alveolar ventilation
Arterial blood pH	**pH**		7.35 to 7.45 pH	Acidosis (pH <7.35) Respiratory (inadequate alveolar ventilation) Metabolic (gain of acid and/or loss of base) Alkalosis (pH >7.45) Respiratory (excessive alveolar ventilation) Metabolic (gain of base or loss of acid)
Alveolar-arterial O_2 difference	A-aDo_2 A-aPo_2		<10 mm Hg breathing room air	Primarily reflects mismatching of ventilation and perfusion and/or shunts; may also be affected by diffusion defects
Dead space/tidal volume ratio	$\dot{V}_D/\dot{V}_T$	Determined from arterial and mixed expired P_{CO_2}	<0.3	Elevated ratio indicates wasted ventilation; i.e., that volume of gas which does not take part in gas exchange
Shunt fraction	$\dot{Q}s/\dot{Q}_T$	Determined from Po_2 after a period of breathing 100% O_2	<5%	Elevation indicates increased amount of mixed venous blood entering systemic circulation without coming into contact with alveolar air, either because of shunting of blood past lungs to left side of heart or perfusion of regions of lung which are not ventilated

FIGURE 5.28 TESTS OF PULMONARY FUNCTION—CONT'D

This figure illustrates pulmonary function tests and comparative values for normal lungs and diseased lungs (obstructive or restrictive disease).

Chapter 6 Renal Physiology

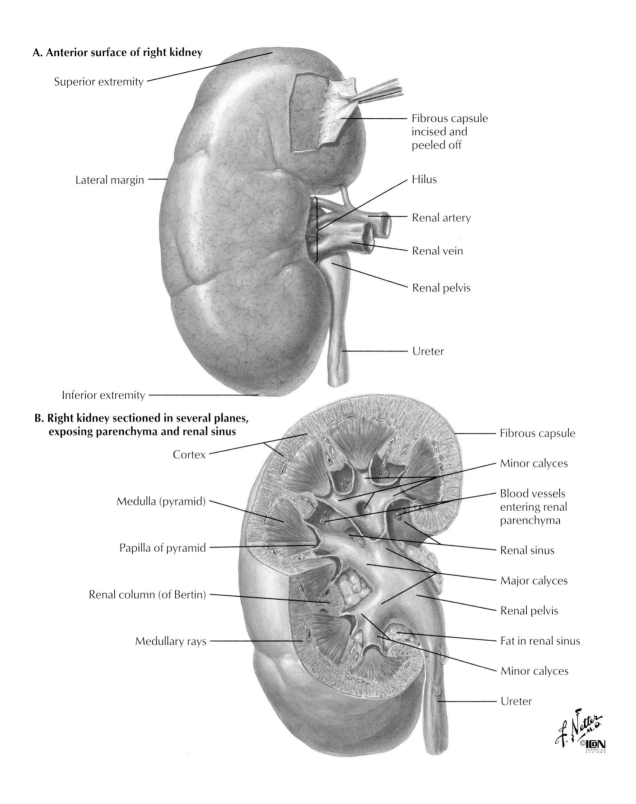

A. Anterior surface of right kidney

Superior extremity

Fibrous capsule incised and peeled off

Lateral margin

Hilus

Renal artery

Renal vein

Renal pelvis

Ureter

Inferior extremity

B. Right kidney sectioned in several planes, exposing parenchyma and renal sinus

Cortex

Fibrous capsule

Minor calyces

Medulla (pyramid)

Blood vessels entering renal parenchyma

Papilla of pyramid

Renal sinus

Major calyces

Renal column (of Bertin)

Renal pelvis

Medullary rays

Fat in renal sinus

Minor calyces

Ureter

FIGURE 6.1   ANATOMY OF THE KIDNEY

The kidneys are paired retroperitoneal abdominal organs at the level of the T11 to L3 vertebrae. They process the blood and participate in the following general functions: (1) regulating fluid volume and composition, (2) excreting metabolic wastes and removing foreign chemicals (e.g., drugs) and their metabolites from the blood, and (3) functioning as endocrine organs. Internally, the kidney is divided into a cortex and medulla, both of which contain the nephrons (approximately 1.25 million per kidney). The medulla forms 8 to 15 pyramids. Urine exits the papilla of a pyramid and collects in a minor calyx. The minor calyces join to form the major calyces and then the pelvis. The renal columns (of Bertin) consist of cortical nephron segments, whereas the medullary rays contain nephron segments that extend into the medulla.

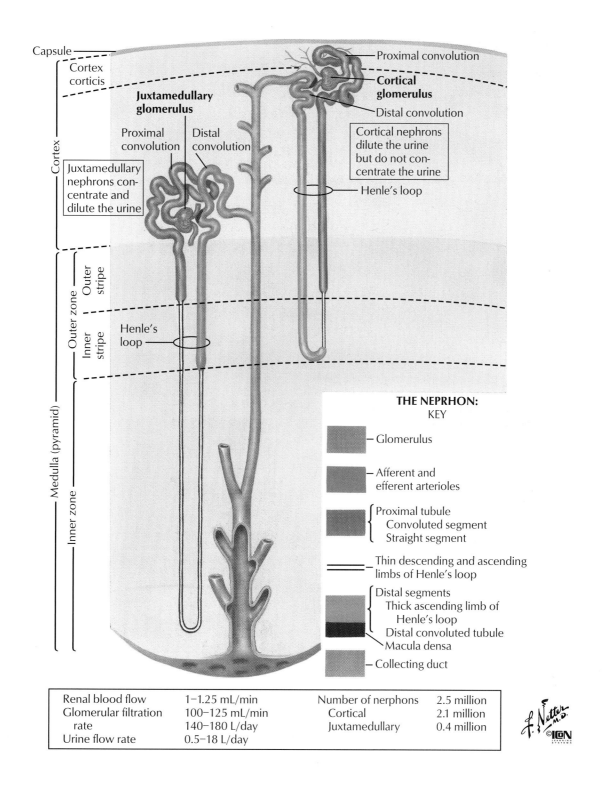

Renal blood flow	1–1.25 mL/min	Number of nerphons	2.5 million
Glomerular filtration	100–125 mL/min	Cortical	2.1 million
rate	140–180 L/day	Juxtamedullary	0.4 million
Urine flow rate	0.5–18 L/day		

FIGURE 6.2 ANATOMY OF THE NEPHRON

The nephrons of the kidney differ somewhat in structure depending on the location of their glomerulus. Cortical nephrons have their glomeruli in the upper or superficial portion of the cortex. These cortical nephrons have short loops of Henle that extend only into the outer zone of the medulla. The glomeruli of juxtamedullary nephrons are located at the corticomedullary junction. These nephrons have long loops of Henle that extend deep into the inner zone of the medulla. There are many more cortical than juxtamedullary nephrons.

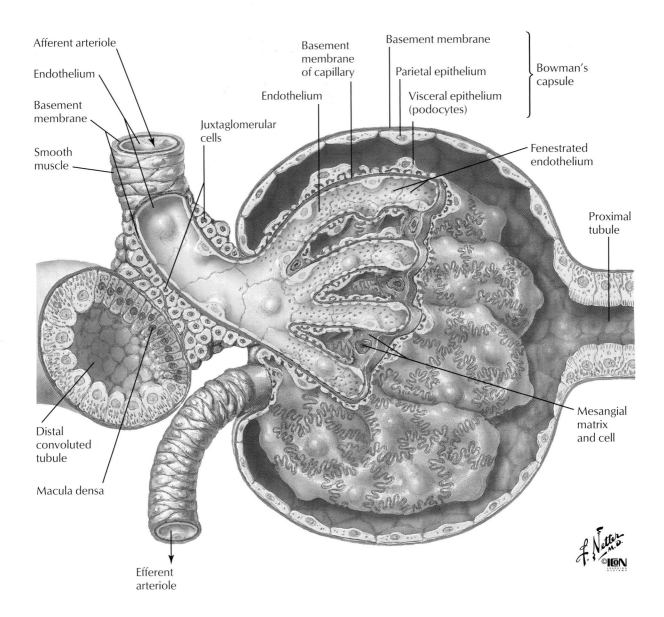

Afferent arteriole

Endothelium

Basement membrane

Smooth muscle

Juxtaglomerular cells

Basement membrane of capillary

Endothelium

Basement membrane

Parietal epithelium

Visceral epithelium (podocytes)

Bowman's capsule

Fenestrated endothelium

Proximal tubule

Mesangial matrix and cell

Distal convoluted tubule

Macula densa

Efferent arteriole

FIGURE 6.3   ANATOMY OF THE GLOMERULUS

Plasma is filtered at the glomerulus. The filtrate is devoid of cells and virtually all proteins (*note:* proteins and peptides that are smaller in size than albumin are filtered to varying degrees). The endothelium of the glomerulus is fenestrated and serves to prevent the filtration of the cellular elements of blood. The basement membrane and visceral epithelial cells (podocytes) prevent the filtration of plasma proteins. The macula densa monitors the delivery of NaCl to the distal tubule and in this way helps regulate renal plasma flow and the glomerular filtration rate—a process called autoregulation.

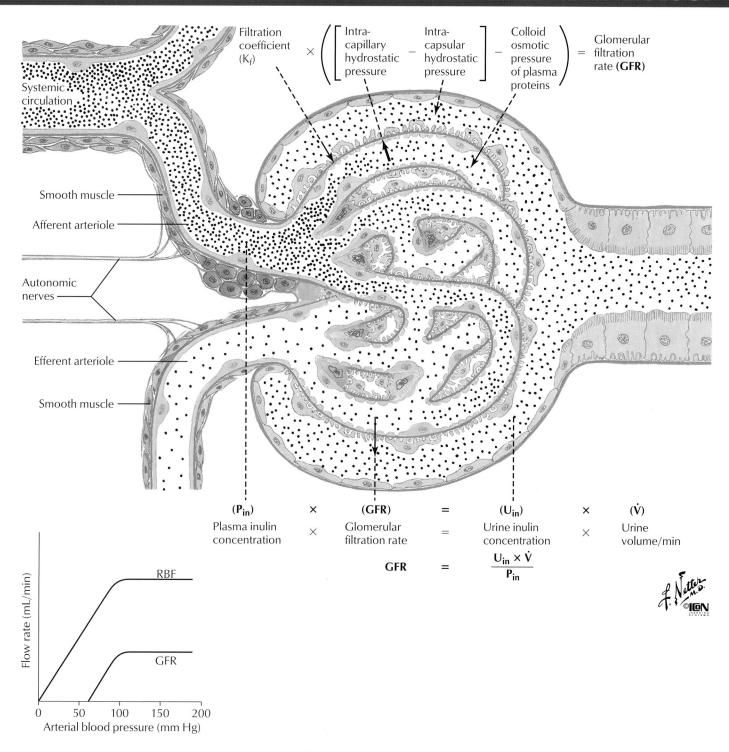

$$\text{Filtration coefficient } (K_f) \times \left(\left[\begin{array}{c} \text{Intra-capillary hydrostatic pressure} \end{array} - \begin{array}{c} \text{Intra-capsular hydrostatic pressure} \end{array} \right] - \begin{array}{c} \text{Colloid osmotic pressure of plasma proteins} \end{array} \right) = \begin{array}{c} \text{Glomerular filtration rate } (\textbf{GFR}) \end{array}$$

(P_{in})	$\times$	(GFR)	$=$	(U_{in})	$\times$	$(\dot{V})$
Plasma inulin concentration	$\times$	Glomerular filtration rate	$=$	Urine inulin concentration	$\times$	Urine volume/min

$$GFR = \frac{U_{in} \times \dot{V}}{P_{in}}$$

FIGURE 6.4 GLOMERULAR FILTRATION

An ultrafiltrate of plasma is produced at the glomerulus. It is devoid of cells and virtually all protein. Small molecules and ions are present at concentrations similar to those of plasma. The glomerular filtration rate (GFR) is determined by the surface area and permeability of the glomerulus (K_f) and the Starling forces across the capillary wall. Intracapillary hydrostatic pressure promotes filtration, whereas intracapsular hydrostatic pressure and capillary colloid osmotic (oncotic) pressure generated by the plasma proteins oppose filtration. The GFR is relatively constant, despite variations in blood pressure (i.e., autoregulation). Changes in intracapillary hydrostatic

pressure are responsible for physiologic regulation of the GFR. When activated, sympathetic nerves constrict the afferent and efferent arterioles, reducing intracapillary hydrostatic pressure and thus the GFR. Although not shown, increased delivery of NaCl to the macula densa decreases the GFR, whereas decreased delivery increases the GFR. A number of hormones can also alter the GFR. Angiotensin II, especially at high concentrations, constricts the afferent arteriole and reduces the GFR. Atrial natriuretic peptide, and prostaglandin E_2 dilate the afferent arteriole and increase the GFR. The GFR can be measured with inulin.

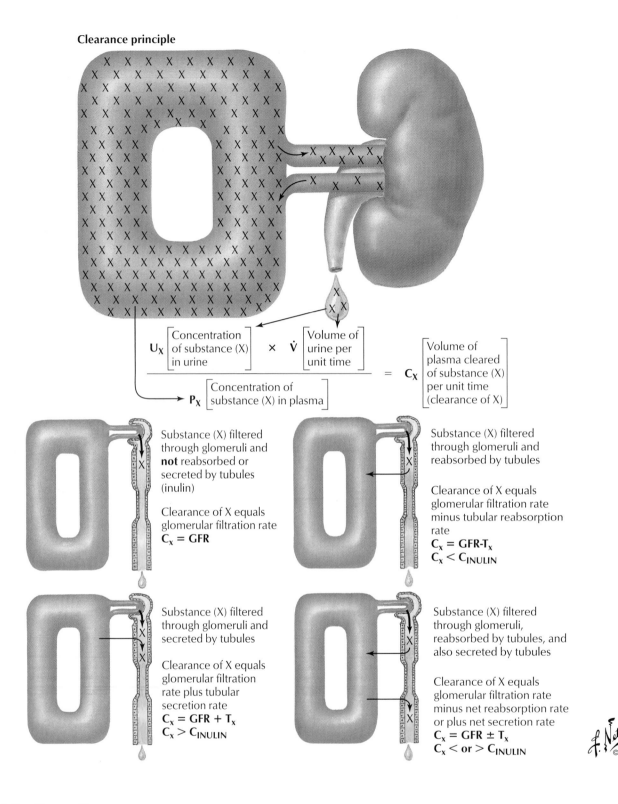

Clearance principle

$$U_X \begin{bmatrix} \text{Concentration} \\ \text{of substance (X)} \\ \text{in urine} \end{bmatrix} \times \dot{V} \begin{bmatrix} \text{Volume of} \\ \text{urine per} \\ \text{unit time} \end{bmatrix} = C_X \begin{bmatrix} \text{Volume of} \\ \text{plasma cleared} \\ \text{of substance (X)} \\ \text{per unit time} \\ \text{(clearance of X)} \end{bmatrix}$$

$$P_X \begin{bmatrix} \text{Concentration of} \\ \text{substance (X) in plasma} \end{bmatrix}$$

Substance (X) filtered through glomeruli and **not** reabsorbed or secreted by tubules (inulin)

Clearance of X equals glomerular filtration rate
$C_X = GFR$

Substance (X) filtered through glomeruli and reabsorbed by tubules

Clearance of X equals glomerular filtration rate minus tubular reabsorption rate
$C_X = GFR\text{-}T_x$
$C_X < C_{INULIN}$

Substance (X) filtered through glomeruli and secreted by tubules

Clearance of X equals glomerular filtration rate plus tubular secretion rate
$C_X = GFR + T_x$
$C_X > C_{INULIN}$

Substance (X) filtered through glomeruli, reabsorbed by tubules, and also secreted by tubules

Clearance of X equals glomerular filtration rate minus net reabsorption rate or plus net secretion rate
$C_X = GFR \pm T_x$
$C_X <$ or $> C_{INULIN}$

FIGURE 6.5   RENAL CLEARANCE

The renal clearance of a substance provides information on how that substance is handled by the kidney. The clearance of inulin provides a measure of the GFR. If a substance is freely filtered at the glomerulus and its clearance is less than that of inulin, the substance is reabsorbed by the nephron. Conversely, if the clearance is greater than that of inulin, then the substance is secreted by the nephron. Figures 6.6 and 6.7 illustrate in greater detail the handling of a substance that is reabsorbed (e.g., glucose) and a substance that is secreted (e.g., *para*-amino hippurate).

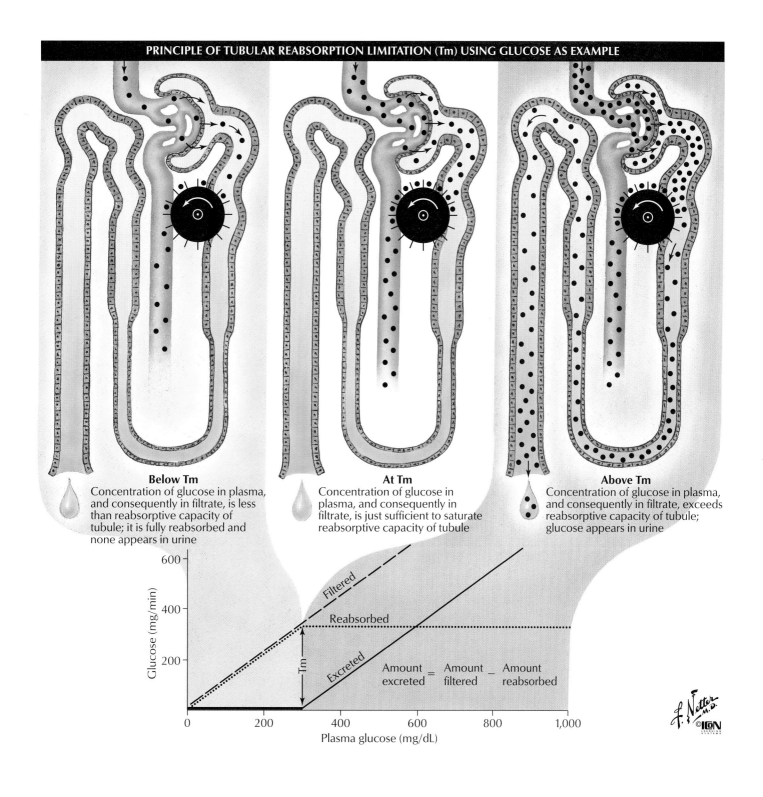

FIGURE 6.6 RENAL HANDLING OF GLUCOSE

Glucose is filtered at the glomerulus and reabsorbed by the proximal tubule. Normally, no glucose appears in the urine because all of the filtered glucose is reabsorbed. However, as the plasma concentration of glucose is increased (e.g., as can occur in diabetes mellitus), glucose appears in the urine. Therefore, the renal clearance of glucose will increase as the plasma concentration of glucose increases.

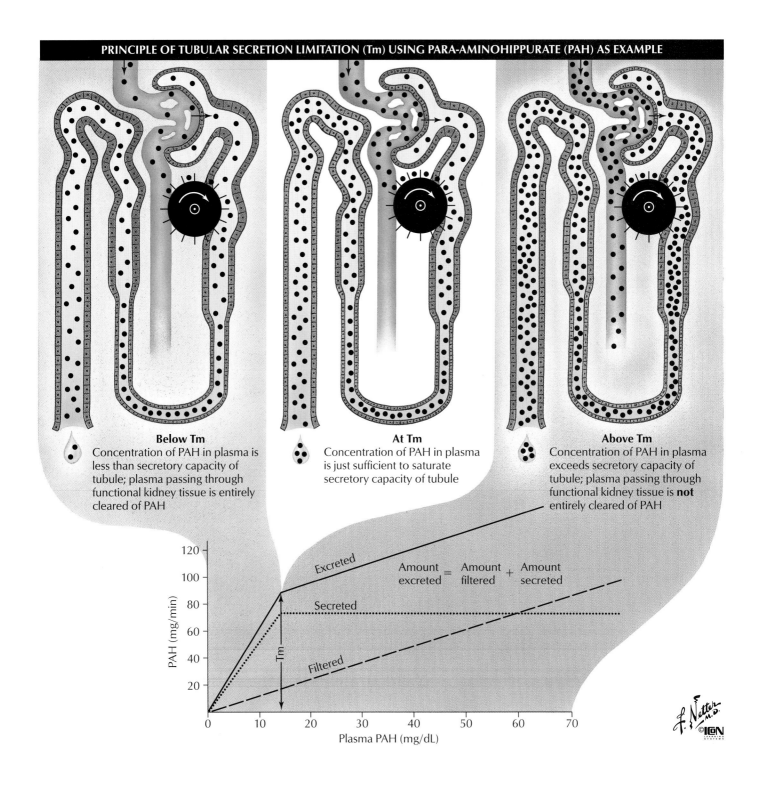

PRINCIPLE OF TUBULAR SECRETION LIMITATION (Tm) USING PARA-AMINOHIPPURATE (PAH) AS EXAMPLE

Below Tm
Concentration of PAH in plasma is less than secretory capacity of tubule; plasma passing through functional kidney tissue is entirely cleared of PAH

At Tm
Concentration of PAH in plasma is just sufficient to saturate secretory capacity of tubule

Above Tm
Concentration of PAH in plasma exceeds secretory capacity of tubule; plasma passing through functional kidney tissue is **not** entirely cleared of PAH

$$\text{Amount excreted} = \text{Amount filtered} + \text{Amount secreted}$$

FIGURE 6.7 RENAL HANDLING OF PARA-AMINO HIPPURATE (PAH)

PAH is filtered at the glomerulus and secreted into the tubular fluid by the proximal tubule. At low plasma PAH concentrations, virtually all the PAH is excreted into the urine. At this point the clearance of PAH approximates the renal plasma flow. As the plasma concentration PAH is increased, the secretory capacity of the proximal tubule is exceeded and the renal clearance of PAH decreases.

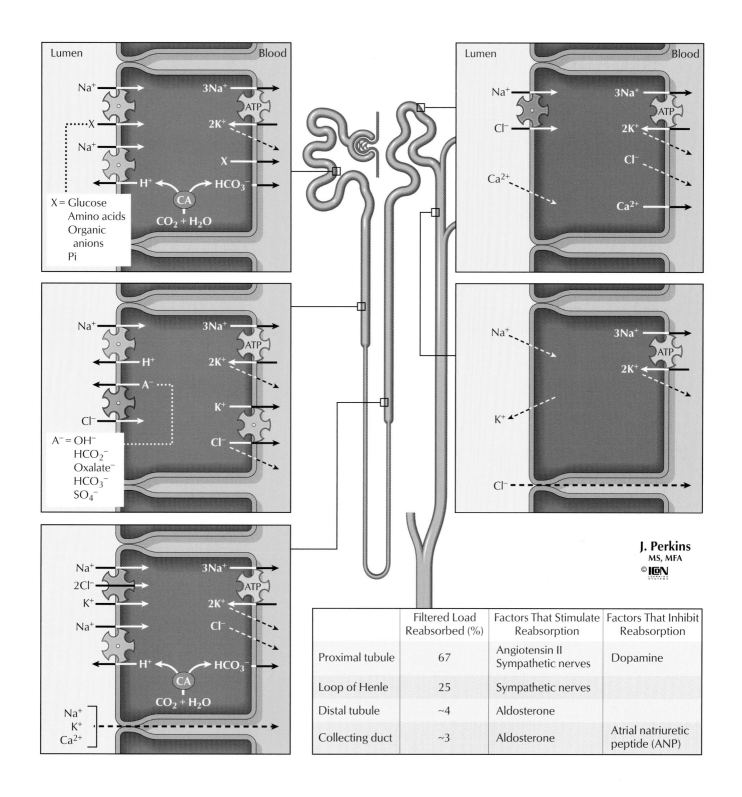

	Filtered Load Reabsorbed (%)	Factors That Stimulate Reabsorption	Factors That Inhibit Reabsorption
Proximal tubule	67	Angiotensin II Sympathetic nerves	Dopamine
Loop of Henle	25	Sympathetic nerves	
Distal tubule	~4	Aldosterone	
Collecting duct	~3	Aldosterone	Atrial natriuretic peptide (ANP)

J. Perkins
MS, MFA
©ICON

FIGURE 6.8   RENAL Na$^+$ REABSORPTION

A large amount of Na$^+$ is filtered by the glomeruli each day. This filtered load (FL) is calculated as follows:

$$\text{FL} = \text{GFR} \times \text{Plasma [Na}^+] \text{ or}$$
$$25{,}200 \text{ mEq/day} = 180 \text{ L/day} \times 140 \text{ mEq/L}$$

Normally, 99% or more of this filtered Na$^+$ is reabsorbed along the nephron (i.e., only 100 to 200 mEq/day is excreted). Depicted here are the primary mechanisms for Na$^+$ reabsorption. Also summarized is the percent of the filtered load of Na$^+$ reabsorbed by each segment and some of the factors that either stimulate or inhibit reabsorption in these segments.

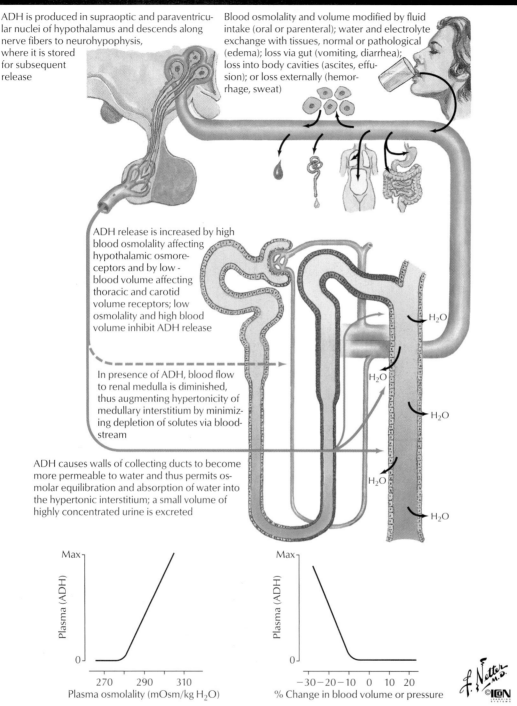

ADH is produced in supraoptic and paraventricular nuclei of hypothalamus and descends along nerve fibers to neurohypophysis, where it is stored for subsequent release

Blood osmolality and volume modified by fluid intake (oral or parenteral); water and electrolyte exchange with tissues, normal or pathological (edema); loss via gut (vomiting, diarrhea); loss into body cavities (ascites, effusion); or loss externally (hemorrhage, sweat)

ADH release is increased by high blood osmolality affecting hypothalamic osmoreceptors and by low-blood volume affecting thoracic and carotid volume receptors; low osmolality and high blood volume inhibit ADH release

In presence of ADH, blood flow to renal medulla is diminished, thus augmenting hypertonicity of medullary interstitium by minimizing depletion of solutes via bloodstream

ADH causes walls of collecting ducts to become more permeable to water and thus permits osmolar equilibration and absorption of water into the hypertonic interstitium; a small volume of highly concentrated urine is excreted

H_2O

Plasma osmolality (mOsm/kg H_2O)

% Change in blood volume or pressure

FIGURE 6.9 ADH SECRETION AND ACTION

ADH regulates the volume of water excreted by the kidneys. Its secretion is regulated by the osmolality of the body fluids and the blood volume and pressure. Changes in body fluid osmolality of a few percent are sufficient to significantly alter ADH secretion. Decreases in blood volume and pressure of 10% to 15% or more are needed to effect ADH secretion. The blood volume and pressure sensors are found in the large pulmonary vessels, the carotid sinus, and the aortic arch. These "baroreceptors" respond to stretch of the vessel wall, which in turn is dependent on blood volume and pressure.

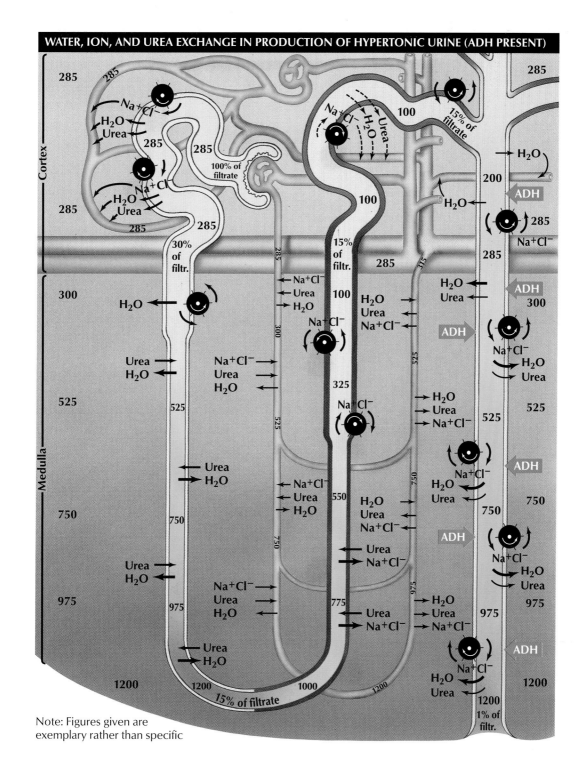

WATER, ION, AND UREA EXCHANGE IN PRODUCTION OF HYPERTONIC URINE (ADH PRESENT)

Note: Figures given are exemplary rather than specific

FIGURE 6.10   CONCENTRATION OF THE URINE

The excretion of a concentrated urine requires normal function of the loop of Henle (in particular the thick ascending limb), a hyper-osmotic medullary interstitium, the presence of high levels of ADH in the blood, and the normal response of the collecting duct to

ADH (i.e., increased water permeability). Under optimal conditions, this results in the excretion of 0.5 L/day of urine having an osmolality of 1200 mOsm/kg H_2O.

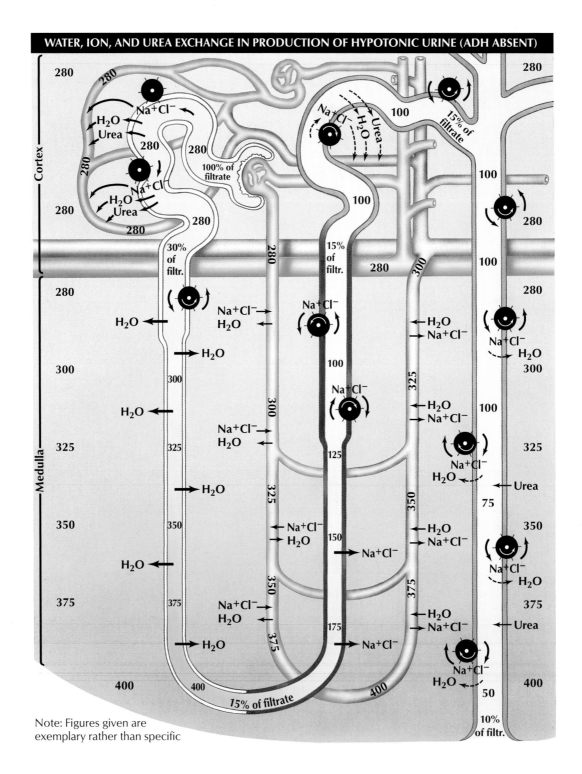

WATER, ION, AND UREA EXCHANGE IN PRODUCTION OF HYPOTONIC URINE (ADH ABSENT)

Note: Figures given are exemplary rather than specific

FIGURE 6.11   DILUTION OF THE URINE

The excretion of dilute urine requires normal function of the loop of Henle (especially the thick ascending limb) and the distal tubule, delivery of adequate amounts of tubule fluid to these segments, and the absence of ADH. Under optimal conditions, this results in the excretion of 18 L/day of urine having an osmolality of

50 mOsm/kg H_2O. Note that the osmolality of the medullary interstitium is reduced. This results from increased vasa recta blood flow (compare with Figure 6.10) and urea removal by the collecting duct.

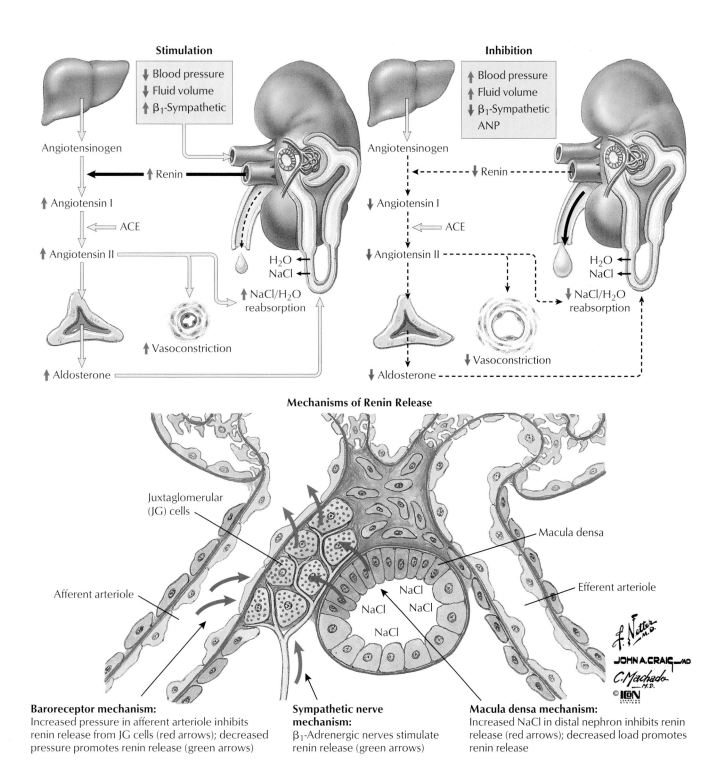

Mechanisms of Renin Release

Baroreceptor mechanism:
Increased pressure in afferent arteriole inhibits renin release from JG cells (red arrows); decreased pressure promotes renin release (green arrows)

Sympathetic nerve mechanism:
β_1-Adrenergic nerves stimulate renin release (green arrows)

Macula densa mechanism:
Increased NaCl in distal nephron inhibits renin release (red arrows); decreased load promotes renin release

FIGURE 6.12   RENIN-ANGIOTENSIN-ALDOSTERONE SYSTEM

The kidney synthesizes and secretes the proteolytic enzyme renin in response to decreased blood pressure and fluid volume (*upper panel*). Renin release ultimately results in increased levels of angiotensin II (AII) and aldosterone, both of which stimulate NaCl and water reabsorption by the nephron (AII acts on the proximal tubule and aldosterone acts on the collecting duct). AII is also a potent vasoconstrictor. Thus, when blood pressure and fluid vol-

ume are low, the renin-angiotensin-aldosterone system acts to restore both. The renin-secreting juxtaglomerular cells are located primarily in the afferent arteriole (*lower panel*). These cells respond directly to changes in arterial pressure, alterations in sympathetic nerve activity, and to the delivery of NaCl to the macula densa. *Abbreviations: ACE,* Angiotensin-converting enzyme; *ANP,* atrial natriuretic peptide.

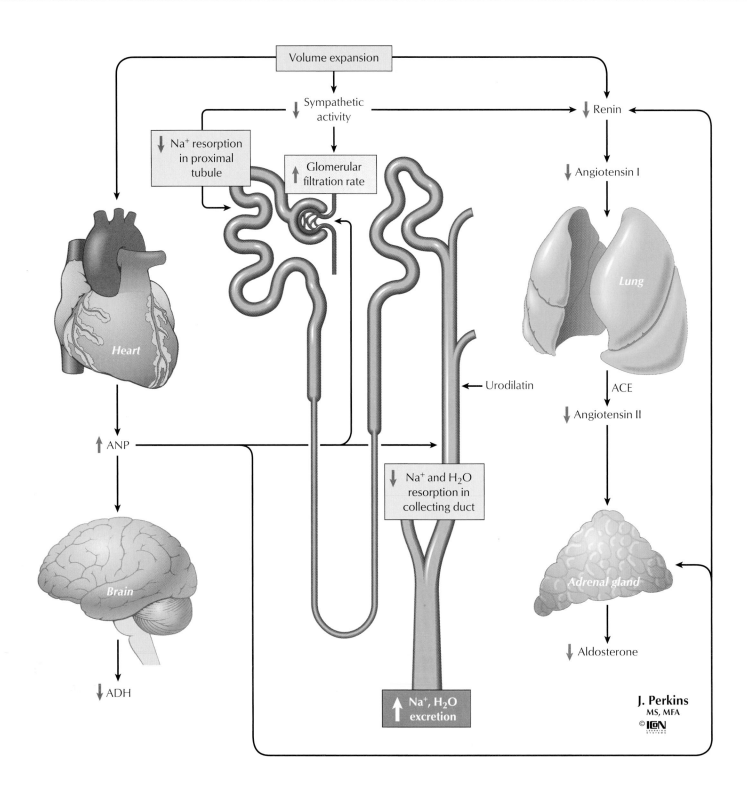

FIGURE 6.13 RESPONSE TO VOLUME EXPANSION

The kidneys respond to an increase in the volume of the extracellular fluid (volume expansion) by increasing their excretion of NaCl and water. The primary mechanisms in this response are summarized. Enhanced NaCl excretion results from an increase in the filtered load of NaCl (increased GFR) and inhibition of NaCl reabsorption along the nephron. This occurs because the sympathetic and renin-angiotensin-aldosterone systems are suppressed and atrial natriuretic peptide (ANP) secretion is stimulated. The actions of ANP oppose those of the renin-angiotensin-aldosterone system. ANP increases the GFR and inhibits collecting duct NaCl reabsorption. The kidney also produces its own natriuretic peptide called urodilatin, which contributes to this response. Decreased levels of antidiuretic hormone (ADH) cause increased water excretion. *Abbreviation: ACE, Angiotensin-converting enzyme.*

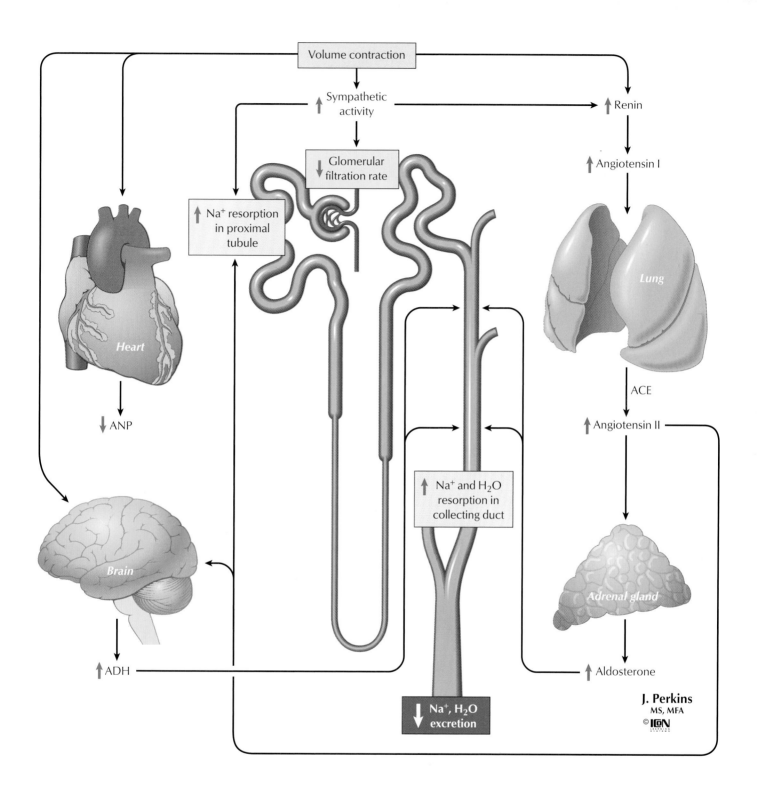

FIGURE 6.14   RESPONSE TO VOLUME CONTRACTION

The kidneys respond to an decrease in the volume of the extracellular fluid (volume contraction) by decreasing their excretion of NaCl and water. The primary mechanisms in this response are summarized. Decreased NaCl excretion results from an decrease in the filtered load of NaCl (decreased GFR) and stimulation of NaCl reabsorption along the nephron. This occurs because the sympathetic and renin-angiotensin-aldosterone systems are activated and atrial natriuretic peptide (ANP) secretion is suppressed. The sympathetic and renin-angiotensin-aldosterone systems decrease the GFR and stimulate proximal tubule and collecting duct NaCl reabsorption. Increased levels of antidiuretic hormone (ADH) cause decreased water excretion. *Abbreviation: ACE, Angiotensin-converting enzyme.*

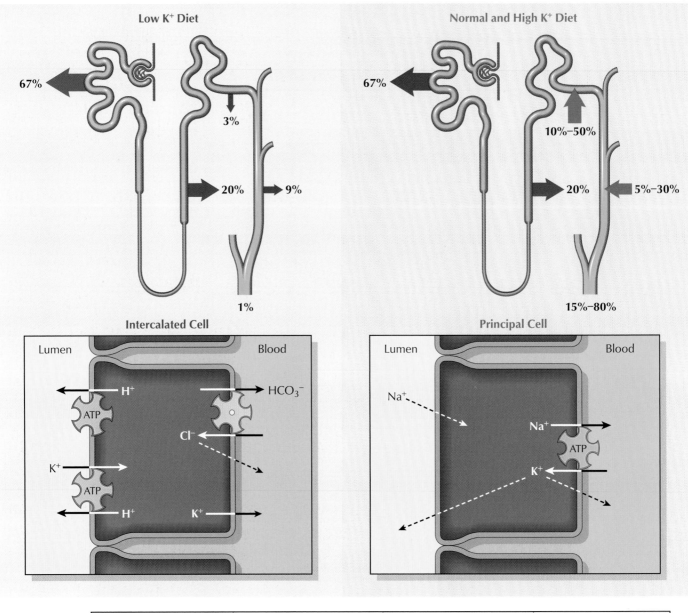

Physiologic Factors That Stimulate K⁺ Secretion	Physiologic Factors That Stimulate K⁺ Reabsorption	Factors That Alter K⁺ Secretion (Stimulate)	Factors That Alter K⁺ Secretion (Inhibit)
Aldosterone Hyperkalemia	Low K⁺ diet	Increased urine flow rate Acute and chronic alkalosis Chronic acidosis	Acute acidosis

J. Perkins
MS, MFA
© ICN

FIGURE 6.15 POTASSIUM EXCRETION

The kidneys are the primary route for excretion of K⁺ from the body, and the amount excreted varies with dietary K⁺ intake. On a low K⁺ diet, only about 1% of the filtered load is excreted. With a normal or high K⁺ diet, varying amounts of K⁺ are excreted. Most of the K⁺ that is excreted under these conditions reflects K⁺ that is secreted into the tubular fluid by the collecting duct. The principal cell of the collecting duct secretes K⁺, while the intercalated cell of the collecting duct is thought to be involved in K⁺ reabsorption during a low K⁺ diet. The mechanisms of K⁺ reabsorption by the proximal tubule and thick ascending limb of Henle's loop are depicted in Figure 6.8, and these are not influenced by dietary K⁺.

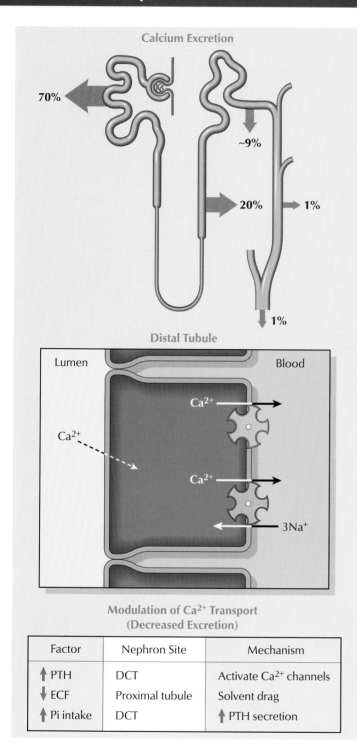

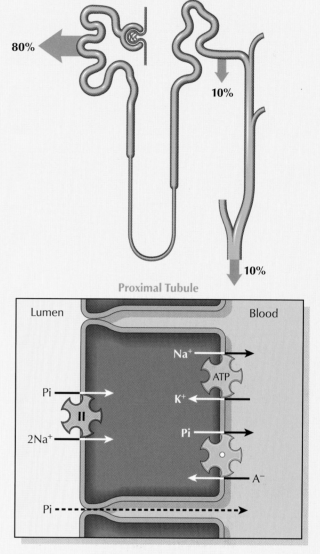

Calcium Excretion

70%

~9%

20%

1%

1%

Distal Tubule

Lumen | Blood

Ca²⁺

Ca²⁺

Ca²⁺

3Na⁺

Modulation of Ca²⁺ Transport
(Decreased Excretion)

Factor	Nephron Site	Mechanism
↑ PTH	DCT	Activate Ca²⁺ channels
↓ ECF	Proximal tubule	Solvent drag
↑ Pi intake	DCT	↑ PTH secretion

Phosphate Excretion

80%

10%

10%

Proximal Tubule

Lumen | Blood

Na⁺

ATP

Pi

K⁺

2Na⁺

Pi

Pi

A⁻

Modulation of Pi Transport
(Increased Excretion)

Factor	Nephron Site	Mechanism
↑ PTH	Proximal tubule	Apical symporter
↓ ECF	Proximal tubule	Solvent drag/symporter
↑ Pi intake	Proximal tubule	Apical symporter

J. Perkins
MS, MFA

© ICN

FIGURE 6.16   CALCIUM AND PHOSPHATE EXCRETION

Calcium is reabsorbed along the entire nephron. Its excretion is regulated by parathyroid hormone (PTH), which acts on cells of the distal tubule to stimulate reabsorption. Changes in the extracellular fluid (ECF) volume also effect Ca²⁺ excretion. However, this reflects changes in NaCl reabsorption by the proximal tubule in response to changes in ECF volume (see Figures 6.13 and 6.14) and is not directed at maintaining Ca²⁺ balance. Phosphate is primarily reab-

sorbed by the proximal tubule. Its excretion is also regulated by PTH, which acts on the proximal tubule to inhibit phosphate reabsorption. Changes in the ECF volume also affect phosphate excretion. However, like Ca²⁺, this reflects changes in NaCl reabsorption by the proximal tubule in response to changes in ECF and is not directed at maintaining phosphate balance.

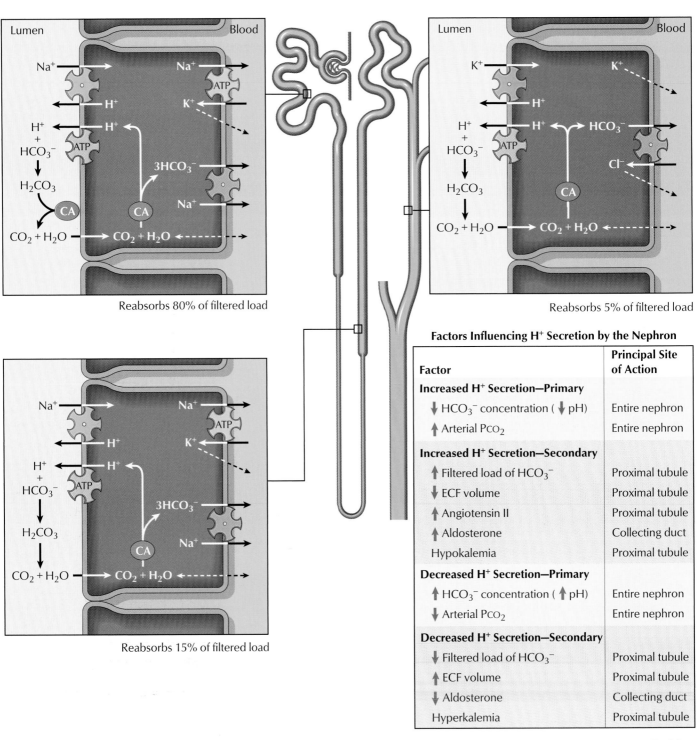

Reabsorbs 80% of filtered load

Reabsorbs 5% of filtered load

Reabsorbs 15% of filtered load

Factors Influencing H⁺ Secretion by the Nephron

Factor	Principal Site of Action
Increased H⁺ Secretion—Primary	
↓ HCO₃⁻ concentration (↓ pH)	Entire nephron
↑ Arterial PCO₂	Entire nephron
Increased H⁺ Secretion—Secondary	
↑ Filtered load of HCO₃⁻	Proximal tubule
↓ ECF volume	Proximal tubule
↑ Angiotensin II	Proximal tubule
↑ Aldosterone	Collecting duct
Hypokalemia	Proximal tubule
Decreased H⁺ Secretion—Primary	
↑ HCO₃⁻ concentration (↑ pH)	Entire nephron
↓ Arterial PCO₂	Entire nephron
Decreased H⁺ Secretion—Secondary	
↓ Filtered load of HCO₃⁻	Proximal tubule
↑ ECF volume	Proximal tubule
↓ Aldosterone	Collecting duct
Hyperkalemia	Proximal tubule

J. Perkins
MS, MFA
© ICON

Figure 6.17   HCO₃⁻ Reabsorption

Bicarbonate is freely filtered and reabsorbed by the process of H⁺ secretion along the nephron. Normally, all the filtered HCO₃⁻ is reabsorbed and none appears in the urine. Changes in systemic acid-base balance are the primary factors that regulate H⁺ secretion. However, a number of other factors can also influence the kidneys ability to secrete H⁺ and thus reabsorb HCO₃⁻.

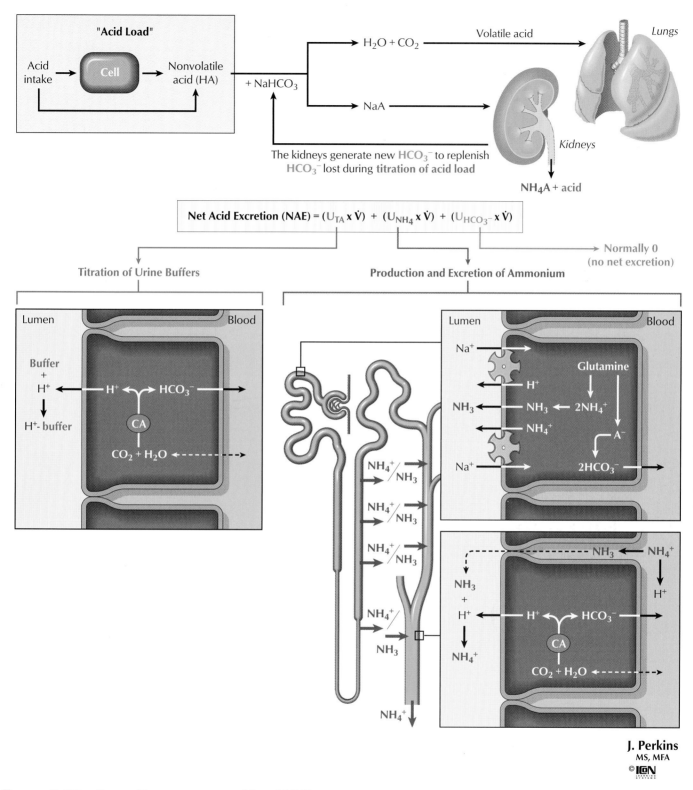

FIGURE 6.18   RENAL PRODUCTION OF NEW HCO$_3^-$

The kidneys generate new HCO$_3^-$ to replenish that which is lost during the titration of the daily acid load. This occurs by the process of net acid excretion (NAE). Normally, the entire filtered load of HCO$_3^-$ is reabsorbed (see Figure 6.17), and none appears in the urine. This process does not produce new HCO$_3^-$, but simply prevents its loss from the body. New HCO$_3^-$ is produced when the kidneys excrete H$^+$ with urinary buffers (the primary urine buffer is phosphate) and when the kidneys produce and excrete NH$_4^+$. The production and excretion of NH$_4^+$ is the most important component of NAE because these processes are regulated in response to acid-base disorders. Acidosis stimulates NH$_4^+$ production (from glutamine in the proximal tubule) and its excretion, whereas alkalosis inhibits these process. Acid-base balance is maintained when NAE is the same as the daily acid load, which is approximately 1 mEq/kg body weight/day. *Abbreviations:* U_{TA}, Urine concentration of titratable acid; U_{NH_4}, urine concentration of ammonium; U_{HCO_3}, urine concentration of bicarbonate; $\dot{V}$ = urine flow rate.

Chapter 7 Gastrointestinal Physiology

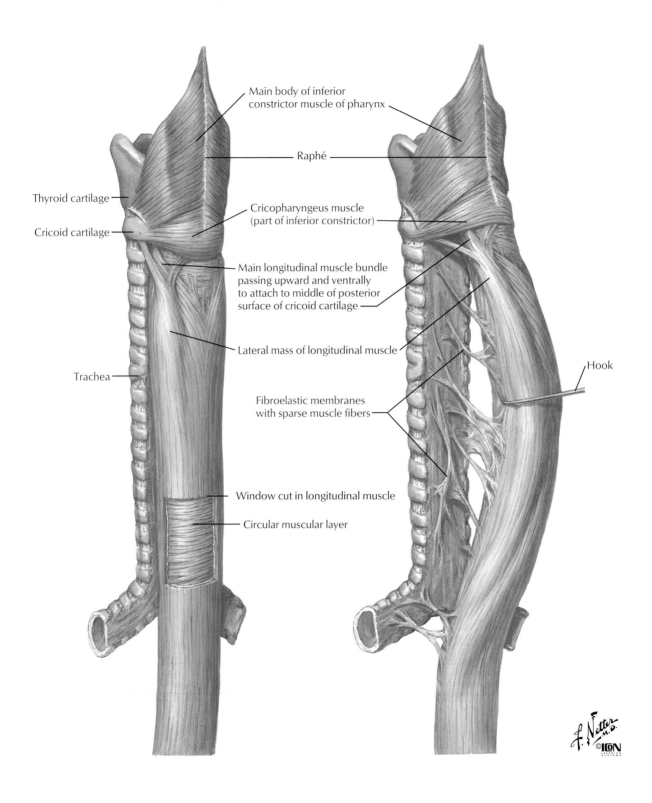

Main body of inferior constrictor muscle of pharynx

Raphé

Thyroid cartilage

Cricoid cartilage

Cricopharyngeus muscle (part of inferior constrictor)

Main longitudinal muscle bundle passing upward and ventrally to attach to middle of posterior surface of cricoid cartilage

Lateral mass of longitudinal muscle

Trachea

Hook

Fibroelastic membranes with sparse muscle fibers

Window cut in longitudinal muscle

Circular muscular layer

FIGURE 7.1 ESOPHAGUS

The esophagus lies posterior to the trachea and extends from the oropharynx to the stomach. It propels food and fluid to the stomach by peristalsis. The muscle of the upper third of the esophagus is skeletal, the lower third is smooth muscle, and the middle third is mixed skeletal and smooth muscle. The muscular walls of the esophagus form an outer longitudinal and an inner circular layer.

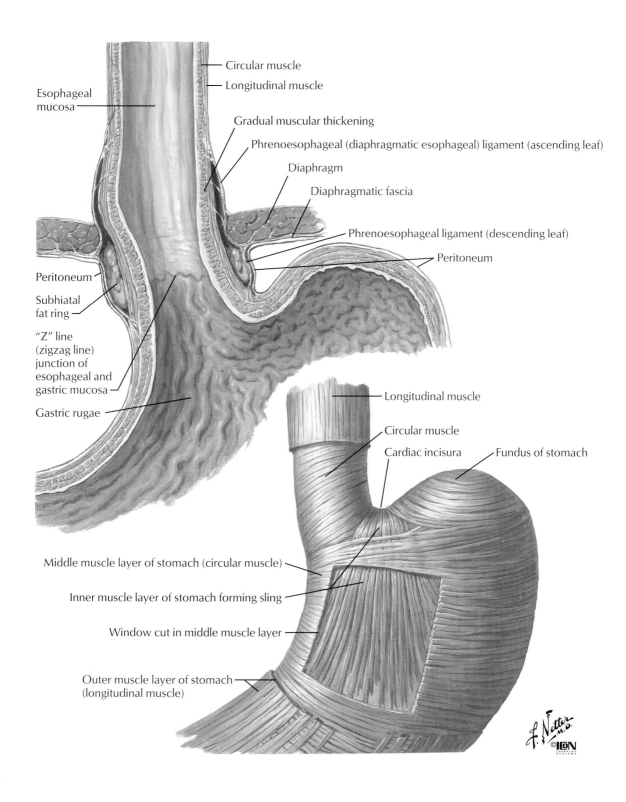

FIGURE 7.2   GASTROESOPHAGEAL JUNCTION

The smooth muscle of the lower esophagus increases in thickness at the junction with the stomach and forms the lower esophageal sphincter (LES). The LES lies where the esophagus passes through the diaphragm, and at this point, the esophageal mucosa changes to gastric mucosa (Z line). The stomach has three muscle layers in its walls, and the most orad, or cardiac, portion of the stomach relaxes (receptive relaxation) to receive the food bolus from the esophagus.

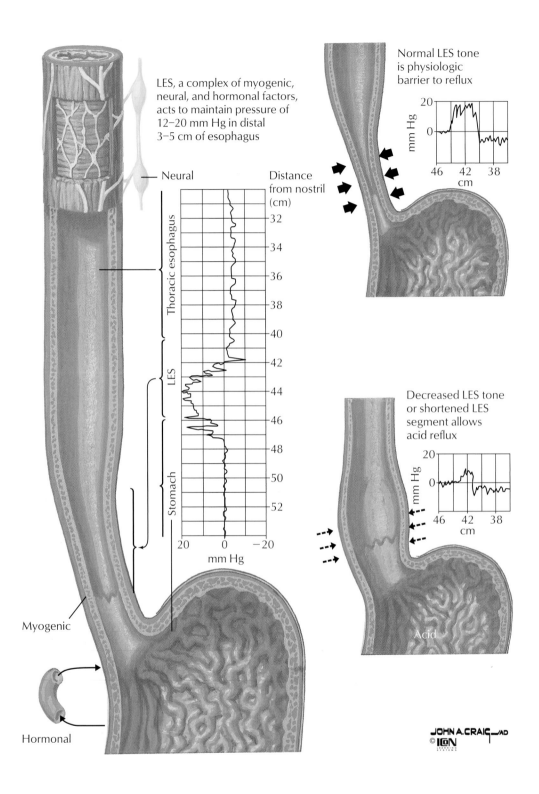

LES, a complex of myogenic, neural, and hormonal factors, acts to maintain pressure of 12–20 mm Hg in distal 3–5 cm of esophagus

Normal LES tone is physiologic barrier to reflux

Decreased LES tone or shortened LES segment allows acid reflux

Acid

Neural

Myogenic

Hormonal

Thoracic esophagus
LES
Stomach

Distance from nostril (cm)

JOHN A. CRAIG—AD
©ICON

FIGURE 7.3   LOWER ESOPHAGEAL SPHINCTER

Peristalsis is initiated by the voluntary action of swallowing, which is controlled by efferent fibers in the vagus. Vagal fibers synapse on neurons within the myenteric plexus (enteric nervous system) of the esophagus. The myenteric plexus directly controls the peristaltic wave by alternatively relaxing then contracting the muscles of the esophagus. The smooth muscle increases in thickness at the junction with the stomach and forms the lower esophageal sphincter (LES). Normally, the resting tone of the LES is high, which prevents the reflux of gastric contents into the esophagus. As the peristaltic wave carries a bolus of food to the stomach, release of nitric oxide (NO) and vasoactive intestinal peptide (VIP) from neurons of the myenteric plexus causes relaxation of the LES, and food enters the stomach.

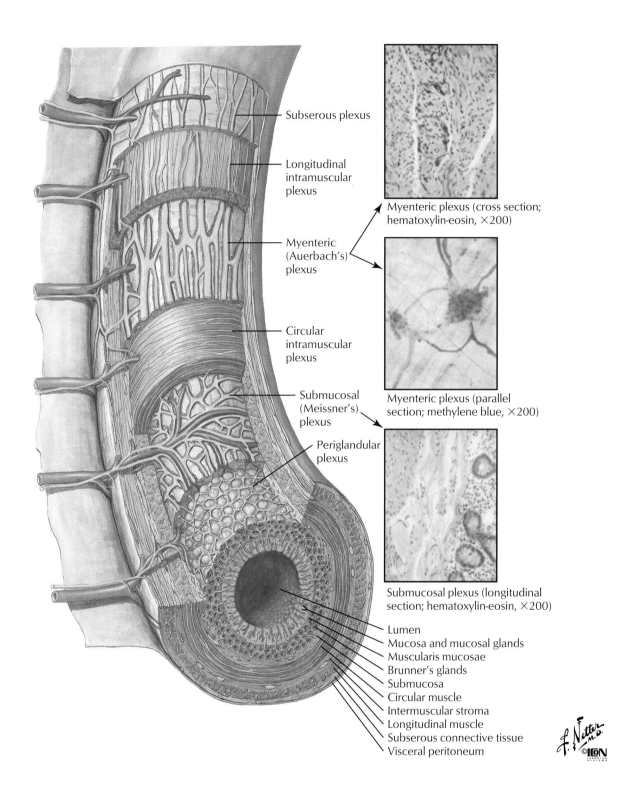

Subserous plexus

Longitudinal intramuscular plexus

Myenteric (Auerbach's) plexus

Circular intramuscular plexus

Submucosal (Meissner's) plexus

Periglandular plexus

Myenteric plexus (cross section; hematoxylin-eosin, ×200)

Myenteric plexus (parallel section; methylene blue, ×200)

Submucosal plexus (longitudinal section; hematoxylin-eosin, ×200)

Lumen
Mucosa and mucosal glands
Muscularis mucosae
Brunner's glands
Submucosa
Circular muscle
Intermuscular stroma
Longitudinal muscle
Subserous connective tissue
Visceral peritoneum

FIGURE 7.4   ENTERIC NERVOUS SYSTEM

The intrinsic innervation of the small and large intestine is by the enteric nervous system, comprised of a neural network in the myenteric (Auerbach's) and submucosal (Meissner's) plexuses. The myenteric plexus is primarily involved in controlling motility, whereas the submucosal plexus primarily controls fluid secretion and absorption. Neurons of this system interconnect with one another and with the neuronal processes of the autonomic nervous system. Transmitter substances (more than 20 different ones have been identified) such as ACh (acetylcholine), substance P, 5-HT (serotonin), VIP (vasoactive intestinal peptide), NO (nitric oxide), somatostatin, and a host of other peptides are commonly found in the intrinsic neurons. For example, ACh and substance P are excitatory to smooth muscle, whereas VIP and NO are inhibitory. Optimal functioning of the GI tract requires coordinated interactions between a host of endocrine, paracrine, and neurocrine substances.

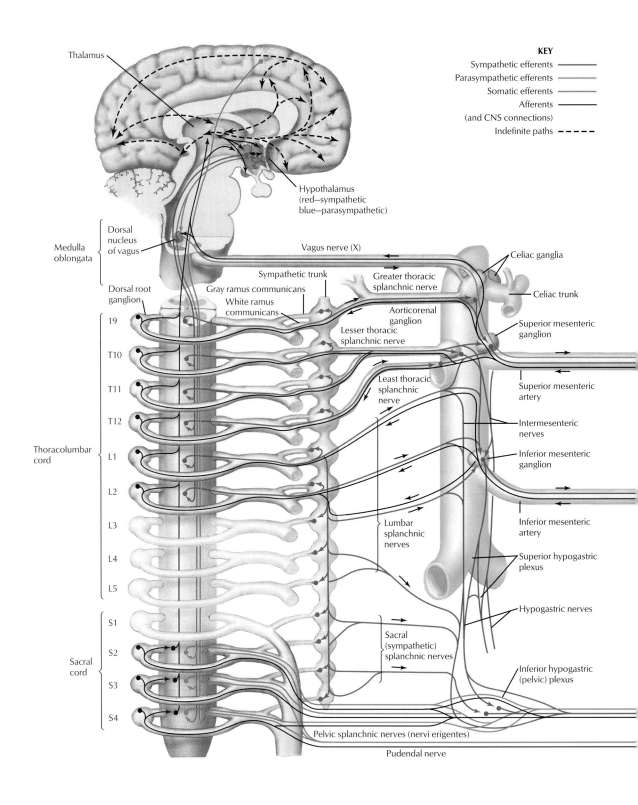

KEY

Sympathetic efferents ———

Parasympathetic efferents ———

Somatic efferents ———

Afferents ———

(and CNS connections)

Indefinite paths ------

FIGURE 7.5   AUTONOMIC INNERVATION

The innervation of the small and large intestines is by the sympathetic and parasympathetic fibers of the autonomic nervous system, which comprises the extrinsic innervation of the GI tract. Sympathetic fibers originate from the thoracolumbar spinal cord (T5–L2) and distribute to collateral ganglia (celiac, superior mesenteric, inferior mesenteric). Parasympathetic fibers come from the vagus and pelvic splanchnic nerves (S2–S4).

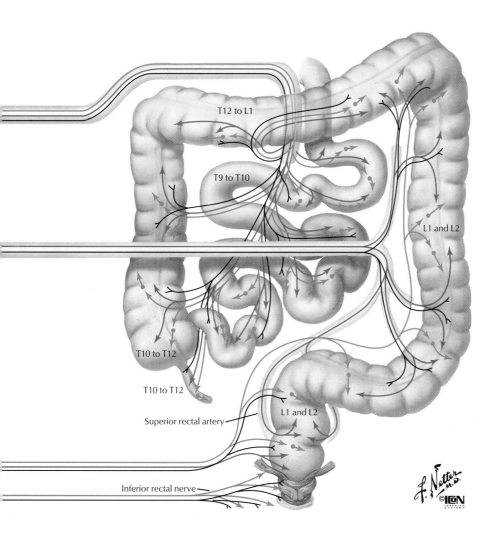

T12 to L1

T9 to T10

L1 and L2

T10 to T12

T10 to T12

Superior rectal artery

L1 and L2

Inferior rectal nerve

In general, sympathetics decrease peristalsis and secretomotor activity (i.e., decreased fluid secretion), whereas parasympathetics increase peristalsis, relax involuntary sphincters, and increase secretomotor activity (i.e., increased fluid secretion). Feedback loops to the central nervous system, especially the hypothalamus and its cortical projections, integrate visceral function and coordinate activity between the extrinsic and intrinsic neurons of the bowel.

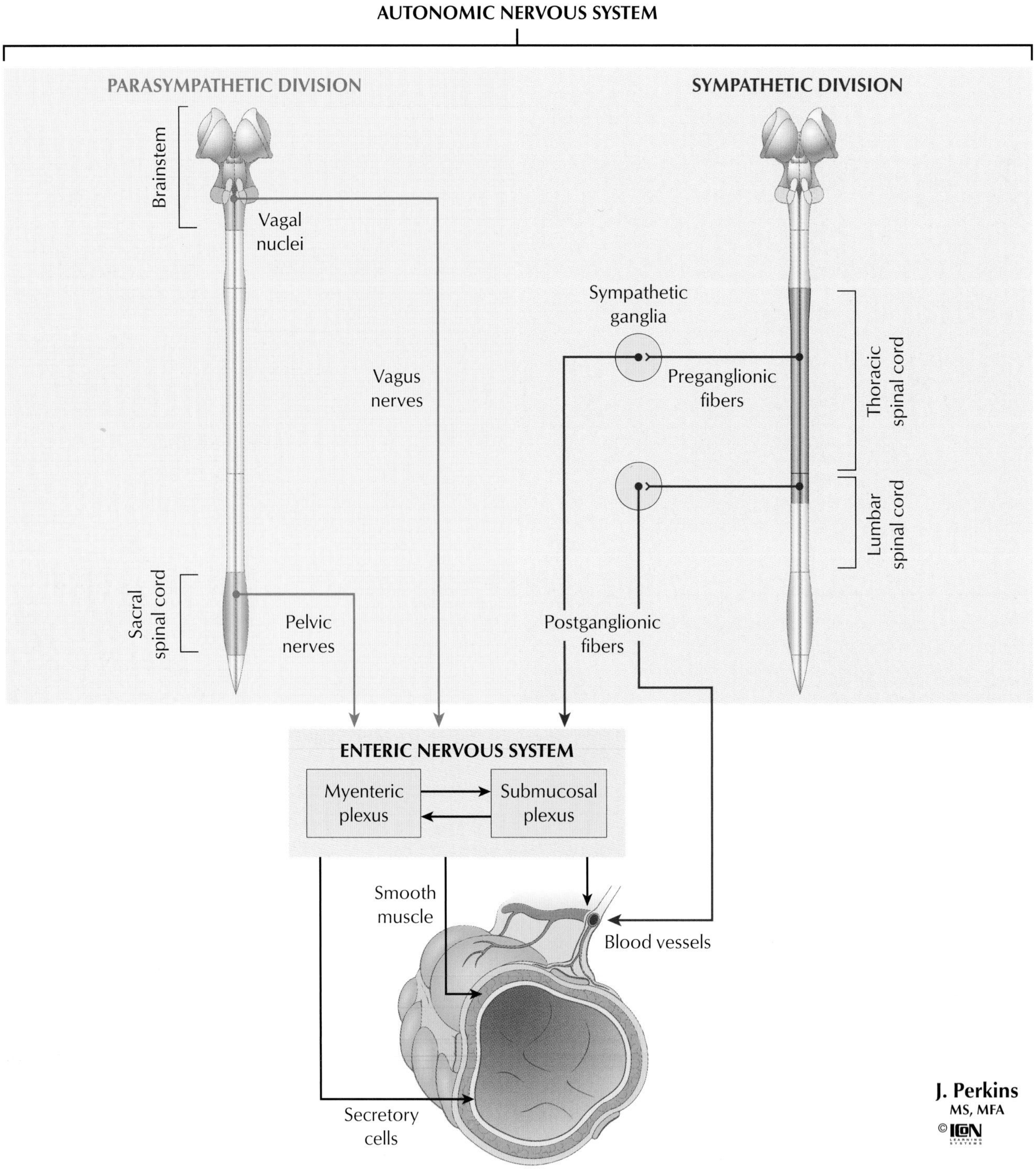

AUTONOMIC NERVOUS SYSTEM

PARASYMPATHETIC DIVISION

Brainstem

Vagal nuclei

Vagus nerves

Sacral spinal cord

Pelvic nerves

SYMPATHETIC DIVISION

Sympathetic ganglia

Preganglionic fibers

Thoracic spinal cord

Lumbar spinal cord

Postganglionic fibers

ENTERIC NERVOUS SYSTEM

Myenteric plexus → Submucosal plexus

Smooth muscle

Blood vessels

Secretory cells

J. Perkins
MS, MFA
© ICN
LEARNING
SYSTEMS

FIGURE 7.6 INTEGRATION OF AUTONOMIC AND ENTERIC NERVOUS SYSTEMS

This schematic summarizes the autonomic nervous system and enteric nervous system interconnections and coordination of gastric motility, secretion, and absorption. The autonomic nervous system, along with the cardiovascular, endocrine, and digestive systems, also regulate splanchnic blood flow both directly and via the enteric nervous system.

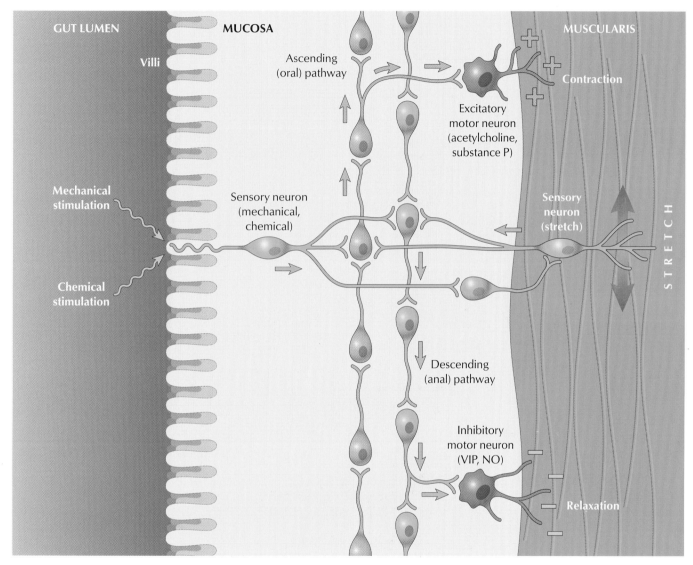

Labels within figure:

GUT LUMEN

MUCOSA

MUSCULARIS

Villi

Ascending (oral) pathway

Excitatory motor neuron (acetylcholine, substance P)

Contraction

Mechanical stimulation

Sensory neuron (mechanical, chemical)

Sensory neuron (stretch)

STRETCH

Chemical stimulation

Descending (anal) pathway

Inhibitory motor neuron (VIP, NO)

Relaxation

J. Perkins
MS, MFA

©ICN

FIGURE 7.7   CONTROL OF PERISTALSIS

The presence of a bolus of food in the lumen of the intestine causes contraction of the smooth muscle above and relaxation below the bolus. This process results in a peristaltic wave, which propels the bolus down the intestine (i.e., from the mouth toward the anus). This process is coordinated by the enteric nervous system.

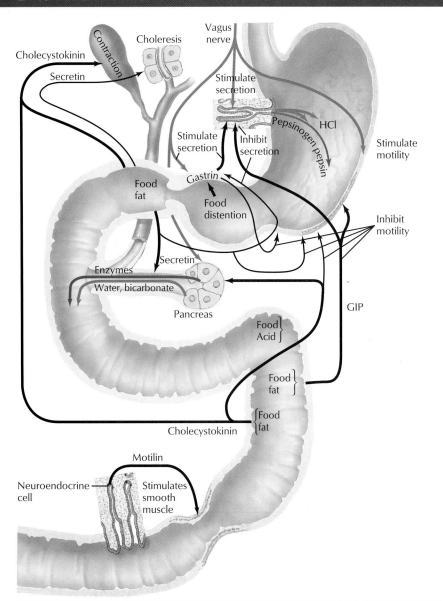

LEGEND

Thick line indicates primary action ━━━━

Thin line indicates secondary action ────

Hormone	Neuroendocrine Cell Type and Location	Stimulus for Secretion	Primary Action	Other Actions
Gastrin	**G cell** Stomach, duodenum	Vagus, distention, amino acids	Stimulate HCl secretion	Inhibit gastric emptying
Secretin	**S cell** Duodenum	Acid	Stimulate pancreatic ductal cell H_2O and HCO_3^- secretion	Inhibit gastric secretion, inhibit gastric motility, and stimulate bile duct secretion of H_2O and HCO_3^-
Cholecystokinin	**I cell** Duodenum, jejunum	Fat	Stimulate enzyme secretion by pancreatic acinar cells and contract the gallbladder	Inhibit gastric motility
GIP*	**K cell** Duodenum, jejunum	Fat	Inhibit gastric secretion and motility	Stimulate insulin secretion
Motilin	**M cell** Duodenum, jejunum		Increased motility and initiates the MMC	

FIGURE 7.8   MAJOR GI HORMONES

The function of the GI tract is controlled by both neural (primarily parasympathetic fibers of the vagus nerve) and hormonal mechanisms. Five major GI hormones have been identified. In addition, a large number of other "candidate hormones," produced by neuroendocrine cells scattered through the mucosa of the stomach and intestines, also play a role in regulating and coordinating GI tract function (not listed). The primary, and some of the other secondary, actions of the five GI hormones are summarized. The "migrating motor (or myoelectric) complex" (MMC) occurs between meals with a period of 1 to 2 hours. It consists of a wave of peristalsis that serves to clean the GI tract by moving residual food particles distally.

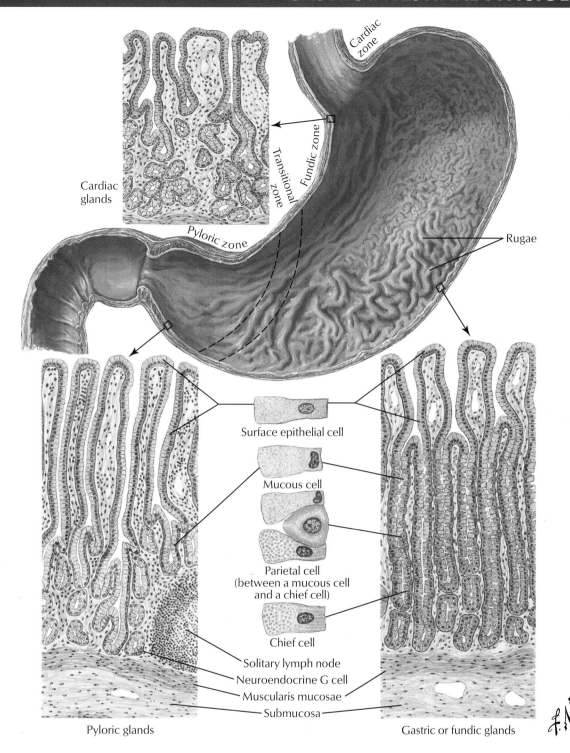

FIGURE 7.9   STRUCTURE OF THE STOMACH

The surface of the stomach is thrown into numerous folds called rugae. The epithelium forms gastric pits with gastric glands at their base; these pits greatly increase the surface area for secretion. The glands differ in structure and cellular composition depending on their location. The cardiac glands are short and branched; the predominant cell type is the mucous cell. The mucous cells produce a watery (low-mucin) secretion that helps liquefy the gastric contents. The gastric or fundic glands are most numerous and form long, straight glands. In addition to mucous cells, they contain large numbers of parietal (HCl-secreting) cells and chief, or zymogen (pepsinogen-secreting), cells. The pyloric glands are branched and are composed mostly of mucous cells. Neuroendocrine cells (G cells) are found in the pyloric glands and are the cells that secrete gastrin. Surface epithelial cells are found in all regions of the stomach. They produce a thick (high-mucin) mucus, which serves to protect the surface cells of the stomach from abrasion by the ingested food.

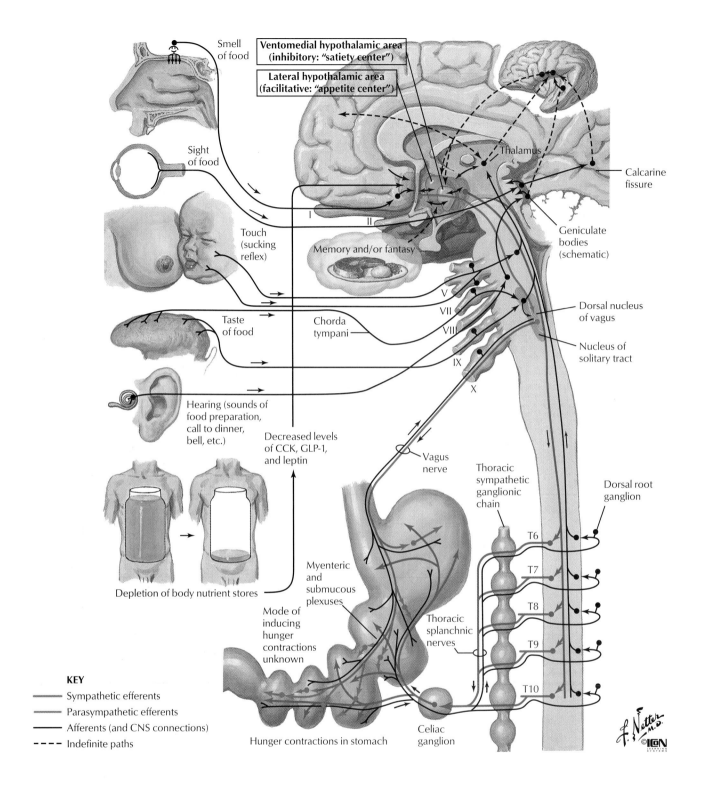

FIGURE 7.10   APPETITE AND HUNGER

The sensations of hunger and satiety are complex and include multiple neural pathways, as well as circulating hormones. Depicted here are pathways involved in the sensation of hunger. Although our understanding is incomplete, the hypothalamus is known to play a critical role in controlling appetite and food intake. When food is ingested, cholecystokinin and GLP-1 (glucagon-like peptide) are released from neuroendocrine cells in the intestine. These hormones suppress appetite and give the sensation of satiety. In the absence of food, the levels of these hormones are low. Long-term regulation of food intake may involve the hormone leptin, which is produced by fat cells. When fat stores are high, leptin is released and thought to act on the hypothalamus to suppress appetite. When body nutrient stores are depleted, leptin levels are low.

Factors Affecting Gastric Emptying

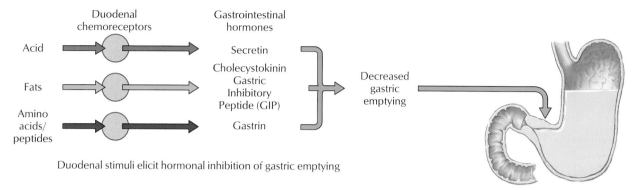

Duodenal stimuli elicit hormonal inhibition of gastric emptying

Sequence of Gastric Motility

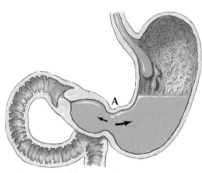

1. Stomach is filling. A mild peristaltic wave (A) has started in antrum and is passing toward pylorus. Gastric contents are churned and largely pushed back into body of stomach

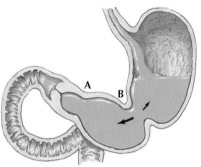

2. Wave (A) fading out as pylorus fails to open. A stronger wave (B) is originating at incisure and is again squeezing gastric contents in both directions

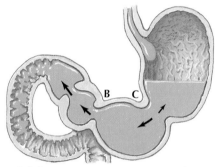

3. Pylorus opens as wave (B) approaches it. Duodenal bulb is filled, and some contents pass into second portion of duodenum. Wave (C) starting just above incisure

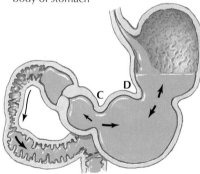

4. Pylorus again closed. Wave (C) fails to evacuate contents. Wave (D) starts higher on body of stomach. Duodenal bulb may contract or may remain filled as peristaltic wave originating just beyond it empties second portion

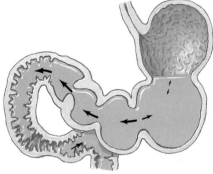

5. Peristaltic waves are now originating higher on body of stomach. Gastric contents are evacuated intermittently. Contents of duodenal bulb area pushed passively into second portion as more gastric contents emerge

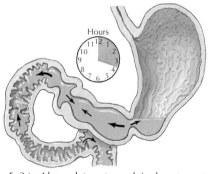

6. 3 to 4 hours later, stomach is almost empty. Small peristaltic wave empties duodenal bulb with some reflux into stomach. Reverse and antegrade peristalsis present in duodenum

FIGURE 7.11   GASTRIC MOTILITY

The motility of the stomach is under neural and hormonal control. As food is swallowed, vagal efferents release vasoactive intestinal peptide (VIP) to relax the stomach. Mixing and churning of the food (chyme) results from contractions beginning in the middle of the stomach and traveling toward the pylorus. Over time, small amounts of chyme are ejected into the duodenum with each contraction wave. The emptying of the stomach varies with the nature of the contents of the food. For example, the rate of empting is starch > protein > fat. Also, solid foods empty slower than liquids. The emptying of the stomach is also controlled by hormones released by neuroendocrine cells in the duodenum and jejunum. These cells monitor the intestinal contents and then modulate the rate of gastric emptying (upper panel).

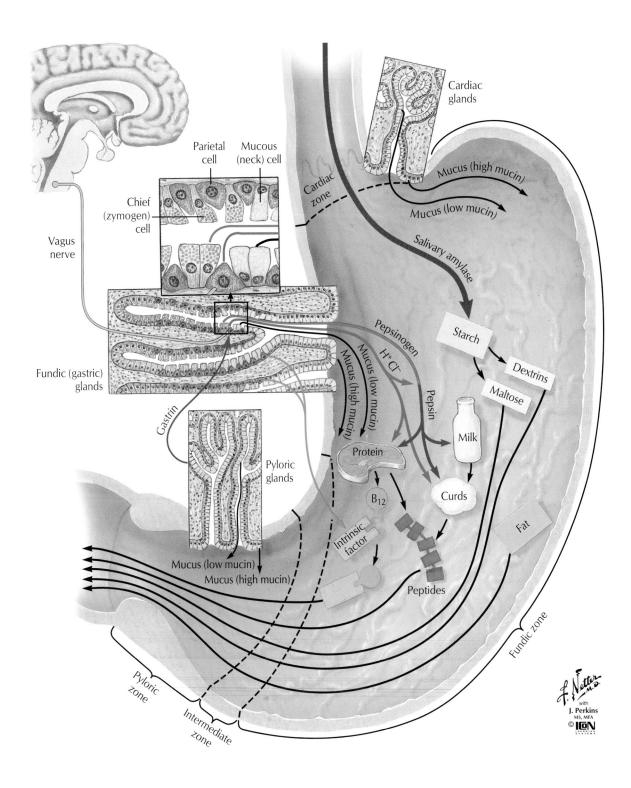

FIGURE 7.12 GASTRIC DIGESTIVE FUNCTION

The stomach serves to break food in to small, more easily digestible fragments. In addition, it begins the enzymatic digestion of proteins through the action of pepsin and HCl. Ingested starches continue to be broken down by salivary amylase. There is little or no breakdown of fat. The parietal cells also secrete intrinsic factor, which complexes vitamin B_{12}. Absorption of B_{12} then occurs in the terminal portion of the ileum.

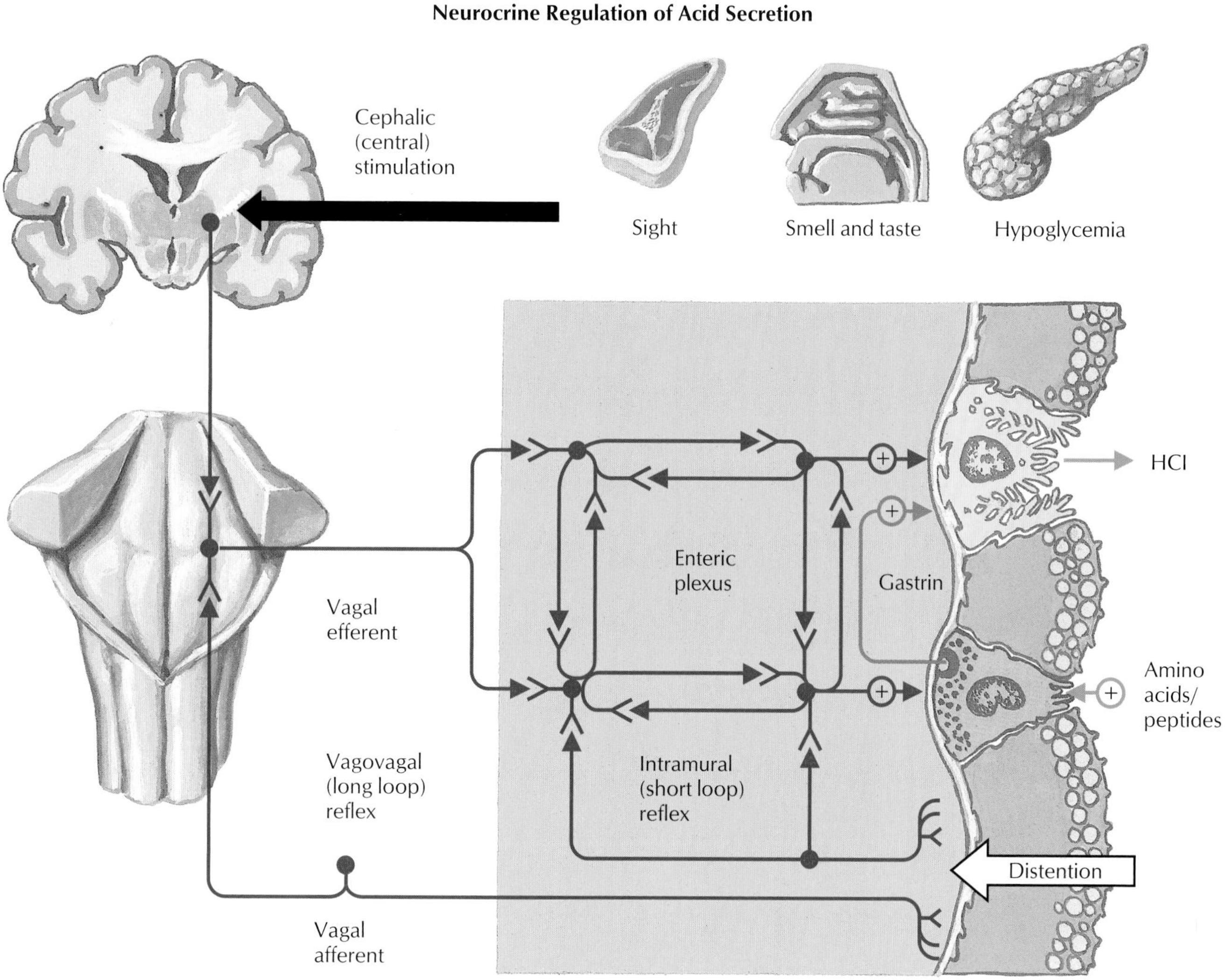

Neurocrine Regulation of Acid Secretion

Cephalic
(central)
stimulation

Sight

Smell and taste

Hypoglycemia

Vagal
efferent

Enteric
plexus

Gastrin

HCl

Vagovagal
(long loop)
reflex

Intramural
(short loop)
reflex

Amino
acids/
peptides

Vagal
afferent

Distention

Gastric acid secretion initiated and modulated by nervous system via central stimulation
through vagal efferents and enteric plexus and by intramural (short) feedback loop and
a second (long, or vagovagal) feedback loop, both stimulated by gastric antral distention

FIGURE 7.13 VAGAL CONTROL OF GASTRIC SECRETION

Gastric secretion, in response to sight, smell, taste, and chewing of food, is initiated and modulated by the vagus nerves of the autonomic nervous system. This initial stimulation of secretomotor activity is referred to as the "cephalic phase." The vagal stimulation acts via the enteric nervous system to initiate gastric secretion of acid (HCl) and gastrin. The presence of acid, amino acids, and peptides, as well as gastric distention, effectively stimulates the next phase of gastric secretion, termed the "gastric phase."

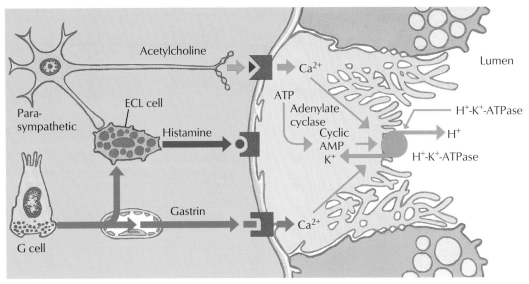

Secretions of gastric acid (H⁺) by parietal cell mediated by neurocrine, paracrine, and endocrine mechanisms. Medical or surgical blockade of these mechanisms affords therapeutic options

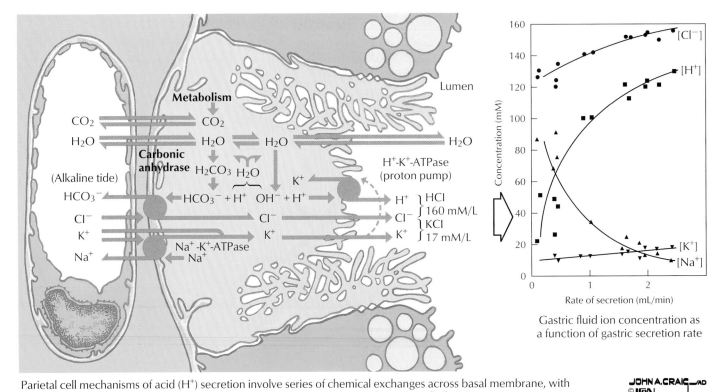

Gastric fluid ion concentration as a function of gastric secretion rate

Parietal cell mechanisms of acid (H⁺) secretion involve series of chemical exchanges across basal membrane, with final active exchange of H⁺ for K⁺ mediated across apical (secretory) membrane by H⁺-K⁺-ATPase (proton pump)

JOHN A. CRAIG—AD
©ICN

FIGURE 7.14   REGULATION OF PARIETAL CELL FUNCTION

The parietal cells secretes HCl via an H⁺-K⁺-ATPase (H⁺ pump). Carbonic anhydrase within the parietal cells catalyzes the hydration of CO_2 and ultimately the production of H⁺. The parietal cell is stimulated to secrete HCl by vagal efferent fibers (parasympathetic), gastrin, and histamine. Gastrin is produced and released from neuroendocrine G cells. The enterochromaffin-like cells (ECL cells) release histamine, which acts synergistically with acetylcholine and gastrin to stimulate secretion. Somatostatin produced by neuroendocrine D cells (not shown) acts on the G cell to inhibit gastrin release.

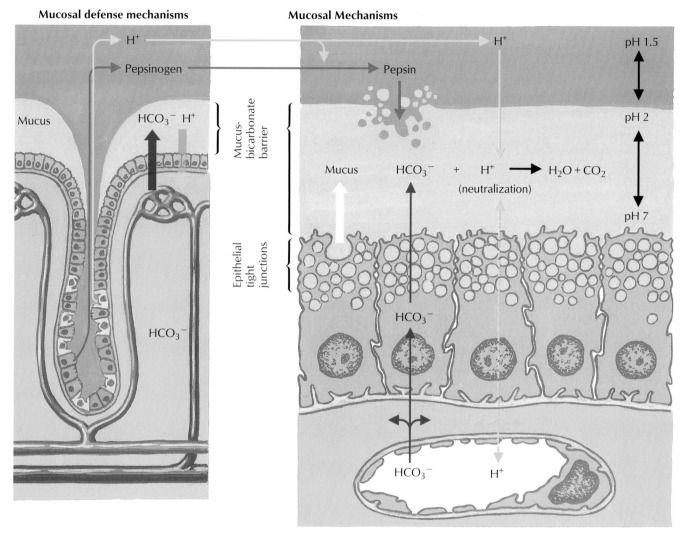

Gastric mucosa and submucosa protected from chemical injury by mucus-bicarbonate surface barrier that neutralizes gastric H⁺ and by epithelial "tight junctions" that prevent H⁺ access to subepithelial tissue

FIGURE 7.15 MUCOSAL DEFENSE MECHANISMS

The high-mucin-containing mucus produced by the surface epithelial cells protects the stomach from abrasion and provides a relatively alkaline environment for the epithelial cells.

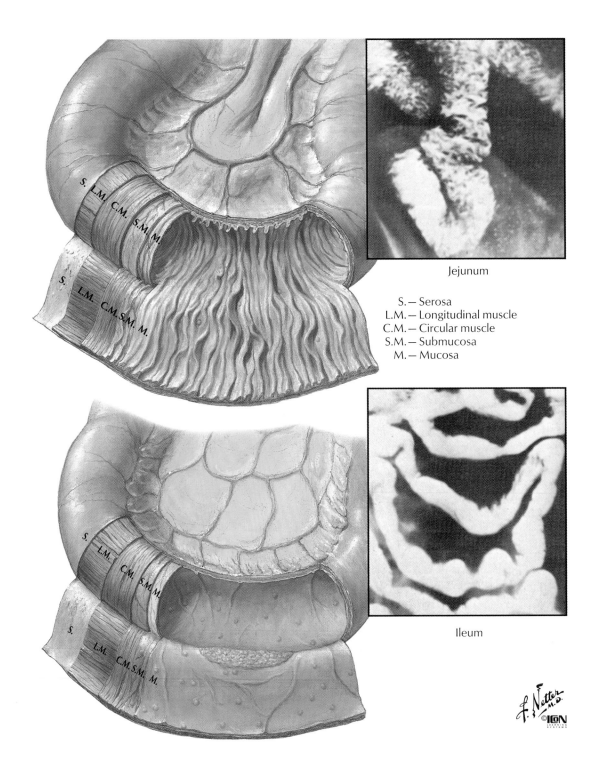

Jejunum

S. — Serosa
L.M. — Longitudinal muscle
C.M. — Circular muscle
S.M. — Submucosa
M. — Mucosa

Ileum

FIGURE 7.16   SMALL INTESTINE STRUCTURE

The duodenum, jejunum, and ileum comprise the small intestine. Anatomically, the duodenum is the shortest segment (about 25 cm long), while the jejunum and ileum are about 6-7 meters long, with the jejunum accounting for the proximal two-fifths of this length. Compared with the ileum, the jejunum has a larger diameter, thicker walls, greater vascularity, less mesenteric fat, fewer lymph nodules, and larger and taller circular mucosal folds (plicae circulares). The absorptive surface is larger in the jejunum as evident in the barium-contrast x-rays of each segment.

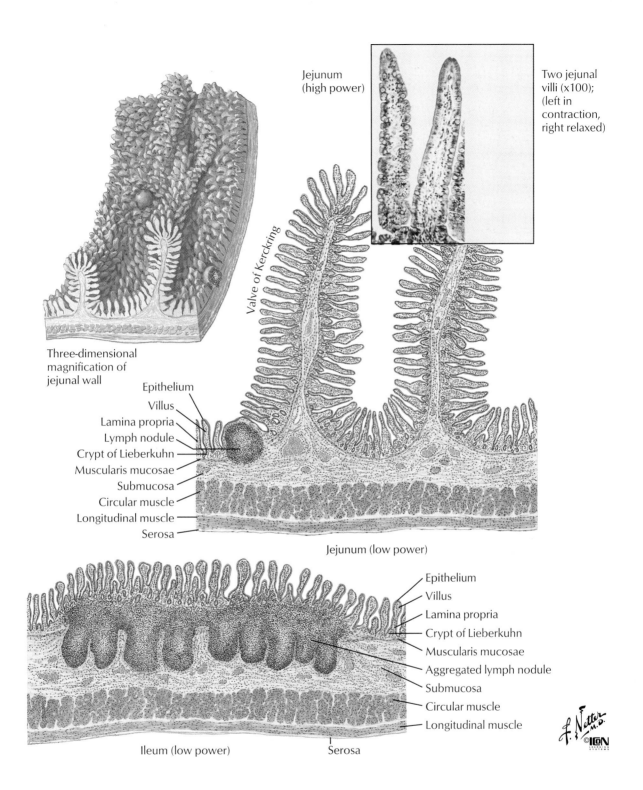

Jejunum
(high power)

Two jejunal
villi (x100);
(left in
contraction,
right relaxed)

Valve of Kerckring

Three-dimensional
magnification of
jejunal wall

Epithelium
Villus
Lamina propria
Lymph nodule
Crypt of Lieberkuhn
Muscularis mucosae
Submucosa
Circular muscle
Longitudinal muscle
Serosa

Jejunum (low power)

Epithelium
Villus
Lamina propria
Crypt of Lieberkuhn
Muscularis mucosae
Aggregated lymph nodule
Submucosa
Circular muscle
Longitudinal muscle
Serosa

Ileum (low power)

FIGURE 7.17   SMALL INTESTINE MICROSCOPIC STRUCTURE

The jejunum and ileum have a large surface area for secretion and absorption. The surface area is increased by presence of circular folds (valves or rings of Kerckring), villi, and microvilli. Because the small intestine provides a large surface interface between the external and internal environments, it represents a first-line defense against foreign antigens. Accordingly, large collections of lymphoid tissue are found in the lamina propria and submucosa. In general, the following changes occur from the proximal jejunum to the terminal ileum; the number and length of the villi decrease, the number of mucous cells increases, and there is an increase in the amount of lymphoid tissue.

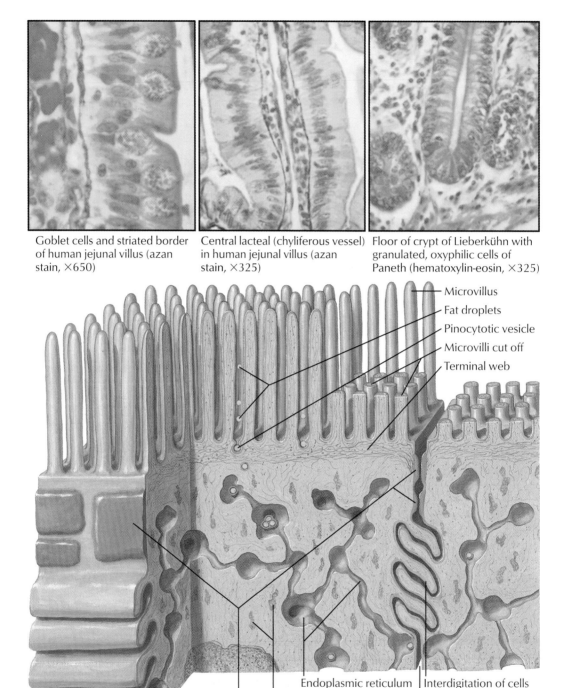

Goblet cells and striated border of human jejunal villus (azan stain, ×650)

Central lacteal (chyliferous vessel) in human jejunal villus (azan stain, ×325)

Floor of crypt of Lieberkühn with granulated, oxyphilic cells of Paneth (hematoxylin-eosin, ×325)

Microvillus
Fat droplets
Pinocytotic vesicle
Microvilli cut off
Terminal web

Endoplasmic reticulum (cisternae and tubules)
Mitochondria
Tight junctions
Interdigitation of cells
Intercellular space

Three-dimensional schema of striated border of intestinal epithelial cells (based on ultramicroscopic studies)

FIGURE 7.18   EPITHELIUM OF THE SMALL INTESTINE

The villi are lined with a single layer of columnar epithelial cells called enterocytes. The apical membrane of the enterocytes contains numerous microvilli. The enterocytes are involved in absorption of nutrients and the secretion of fluid into the intestinal lumen. Interspersed among the enterocytes are goblet cells, which secrete mucus. The crypts of Lieberkuhn are located at the base of the villi and are the site where actively dividing cells are found. The newly formed cells migrate up the villus over the course of 3 to 5 days and are sloughed into the lumen. The crypts also contain Paneth cells, which secrete the antibacterial enzyme lysozyme.

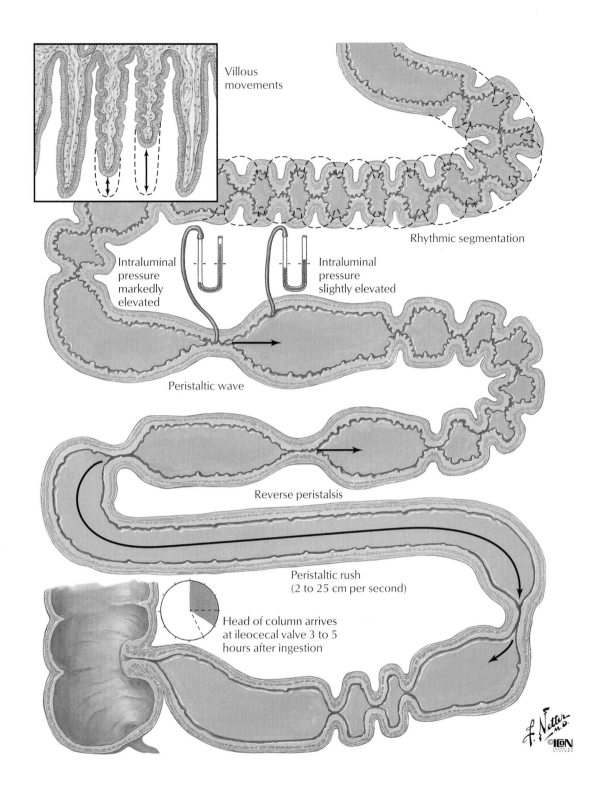

Villous movements

Rhythmic segmentation

Intraluminal pressure markedly elevated

Intraluminal pressure slightly elevated

Peristaltic wave

Reverse peristalsis

Peristaltic rush
(2 to 25 cm per second)

Head of column arrives at ileocecal valve 3 to 5 hours after ingestion

FIGURE 7.19 MOTILITY OF THE SMALL INTESTINE

The small intestine has two general types of motility patterns. These motility patterns are under the control of the enteric nervous system (primarily the myenteric plexus). The first pattern, segmentation, serves to mix and churn the luminal contents. The second pattern, peristalsis, serves to move the luminal contents distally. In some instances, reverse peristalsis occurs, as does a peristaltic rush. In the absence of food (interdigestive phase), there is a periodic wave (every 1 to 2 hours) of peristalsis that begins in the stomach and sweeps down the length of the small intestine. This wave is called the migrating motor (or myoelectric) complex (MMC) and serves to clean the intestine and maintain a low bacterial count in the small intestine. The MMC is modulated by motilin.

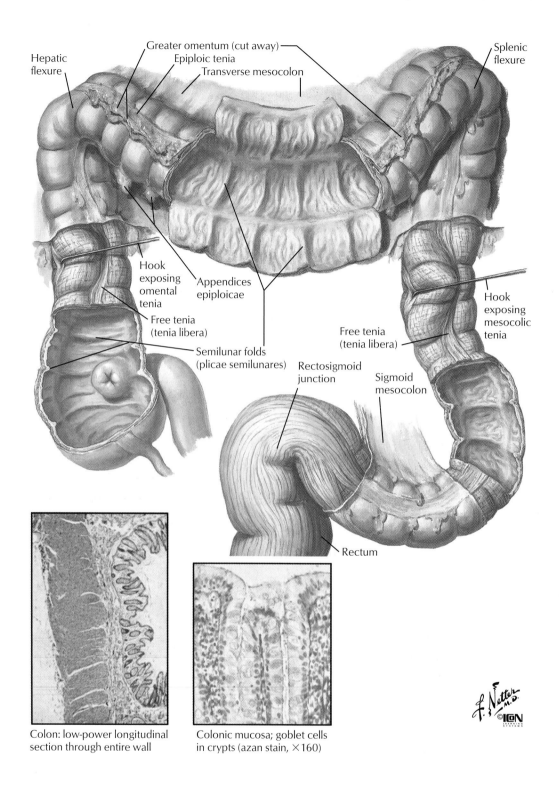

Colon: low-power longitudinal section through entire wall

Colonic mucosa; goblet cells in crypts (azan stain, ×160)

FIGURE 7.20 LARGE INTESTINE STRUCTURE

The large intestine serves primarily to reabsorb water and electrolytes from the feces and to store the feces until they are eliminated from the body. The large intestine consists of the cecum, appendix, colon, rectum, and anal canal. Like the small intestine, the large intestine has two smooth muscle layers, but the outer longitudinal muscle is organized into three thickened bands (teniae coli) that run from the cecum to the rectum. The colon is subdivided into a retroperitoneal ascending colon, a transverse colon tethered by a mesentery, a retroperitoneal descending colon, and a mesenteric sigmoid colon. A large number of mucus-producing goblet cells are found in the colon. They produce a copious amount of mucus for lubrication.

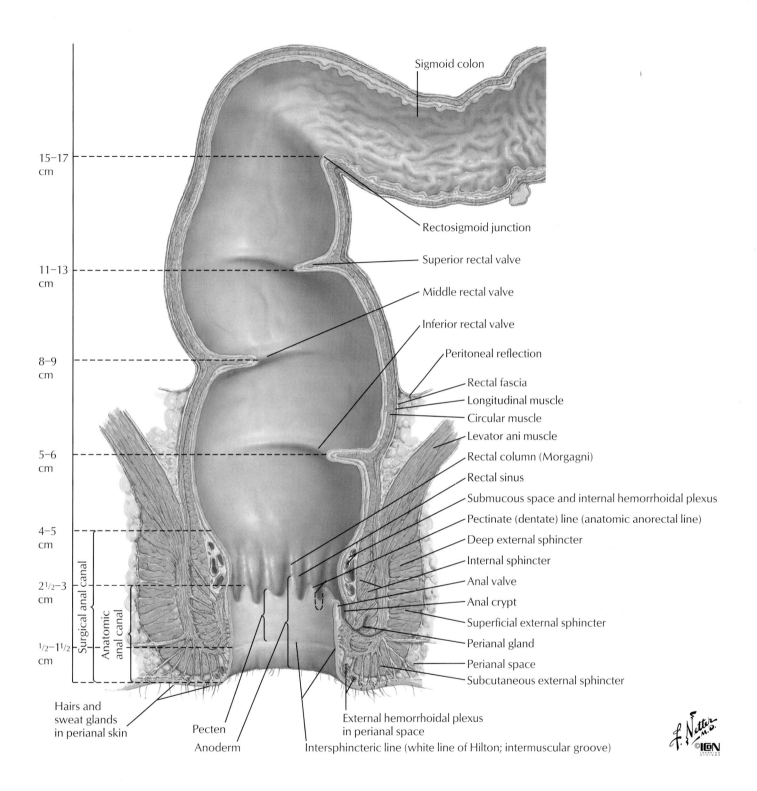

Sigmoid colon

Rectosigmoid junction

Superior rectal valve

Middle rectal valve

Inferior rectal valve

Peritoneal reflection

Rectal fascia

Longitudinal muscle

Circular muscle

Levator ani muscle

Rectal column (Morgagni)

Rectal sinus

Submucous space and internal hemorrhoidal plexus

Pectinate (dentate) line (anatomic anorectal line)

Deep external sphincter

Internal sphincter

Anal valve

Anal crypt

Superficial external sphincter

Perianal gland

Perianal space

Subcutaneous external sphincter

15–17 cm

11–13 cm

8–9 cm

5–6 cm

4–5 cm

2½–3 cm

½–1½ cm

Surgical anal canal

Anatomic anal canal

Hairs and sweat glands in perianal skin

Pecten

Anoderm

External hemorrhoidal plexus in perianal space

Intersphincteric line (white line of Hilton; intermuscular groove)

FIGURE 7.21   STRUCTURE OF THE RECTUM AND ANAL CANAL

The terminal end of the large intestine is the rectum and anal canal. Normally, the anal canal is closed due to the tonic contraction of the internal (smooth muscle) and external (skeletal muscle) anal sphincters. When the rectum is distended by fecal material, the internal sphincter relaxes but defecation does not occur until the voluntary external sphincter is relaxed and the muscles of the distal colon and rectum contract.

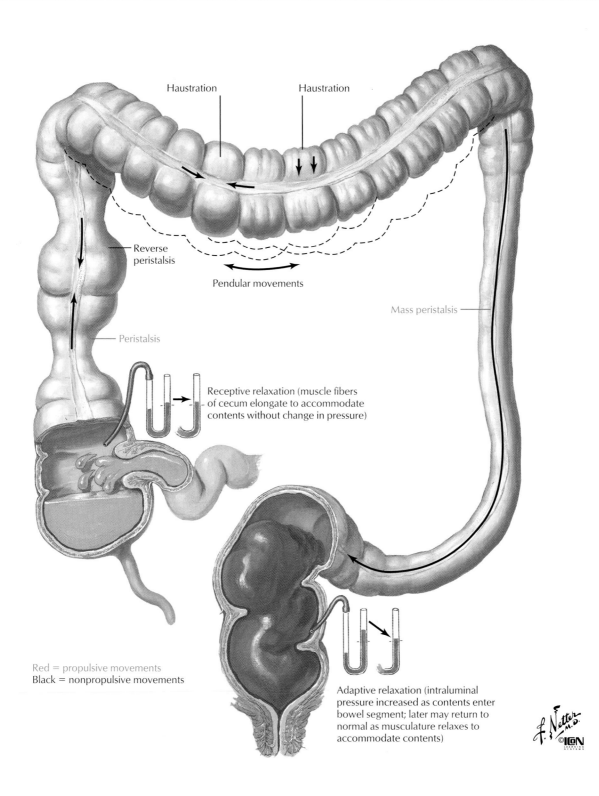

Haustration

Haustration

Reverse peristalsis

Pendular movements

Mass peristalsis

Peristalsis

Receptive relaxation (muscle fibers of cecum elongate to accommodate contents without change in pressure)

Red = propulsive movements
Black = nonpropulsive movements

Adaptive relaxation (intraluminal pressure increased as contents enter bowel segment; later may return to normal as musculature relaxes to accommodate contents)

FIGURE 7.22 COLONIC MOTILITY

Motility patterns in the colon include those that propel luminal contents toward the rectum (i.e., peristalsis and mass peristalsis) and those that prolong contact of the luminal contents with the absorptive epithelial cells. These later patterns allow sufficient contact time for maximal absorption of fluid from the feces. Conditions that promote the propulsive patterns result in diarrhea.

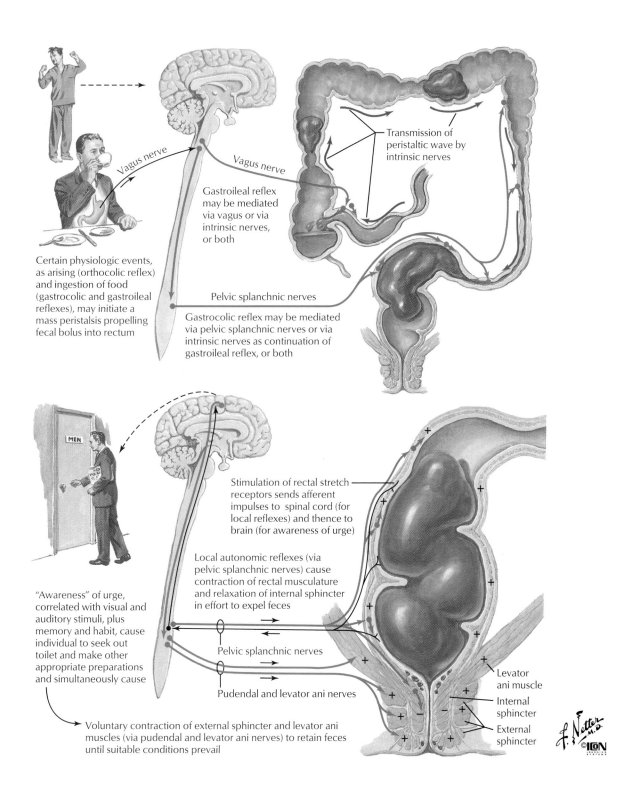

Transmission of peristaltic wave by intrinsic nerves

Certain physiologic events, as arising (orthocolic reflex) and ingestion of food (gastrocolic and gastroileal reflexes), may initiate a mass peristalsis propelling fecal bolus into rectum

Gastroileal reflex may be mediated via vagus or via intrinsic nerves, or both

Vagus nerve

Vagus nerve

Pelvic splanchnic nerves

Gastrocolic reflex may be mediated via pelvic splanchnic nerves or via intrinsic nerves as continuation of gastroileal reflex, or both

Stimulation of rectal stretch receptors sends afferent impulses to spinal cord (for local reflexes) and thence to brain (for awareness of urge)

Local autonomic reflexes (via pelvic splanchnic nerves) cause contraction of rectal musculature and relaxation of internal sphincter in effort to expel feces

"Awareness" of urge, correlated with visual and auditory stimuli, plus memory and habit, cause individual to seek out toilet and make other appropriate preparations and simultaneously cause

Pelvic splanchnic nerves

Pudendal and levator ani nerves

Voluntary contraction of external sphincter and levator ani muscles (via pudendal and levator ani nerves) to retain feces until suitable conditions prevail

Levator ani muscle

Internal sphincter

External sphincter

FIGURE 7.23 DEFECATION

Defecation involves heeding the rectosphincteric reflex and relaxation of both the involuntary internal anal sphincter (innervated by the pelvic splanchnic nerves of the parasympathetic division of the autonomic nervous system) and voluntary external anal sphincter (innervated by the somatic pudendal nerve). Contraction of the distal colon and rectum expels the feces.

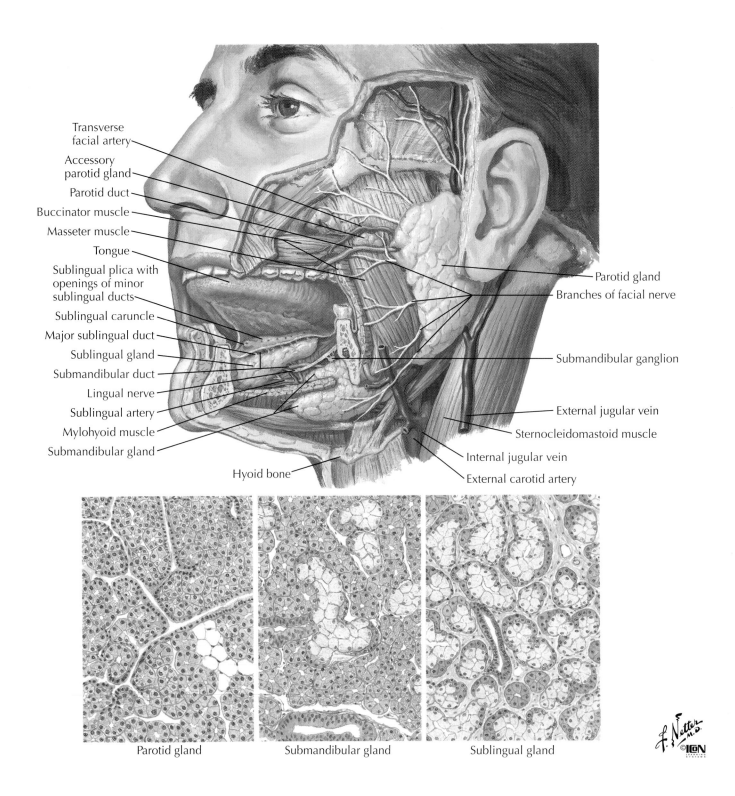

Transverse facial artery
Accessory parotid gland
Parotid duct
Buccinator muscle
Masseter muscle
Tongue
Sublingual plica with openings of minor sublingual ducts
Sublingual caruncle
Major sublingual duct
Sublingual gland
Submandibular duct
Lingual nerve
Sublingual artery
Mylohyoid muscle
Submandibular gland
Hyoid bone

Parotid gland
Branches of facial nerve
Submandibular ganglion
External jugular vein
Sternocleidomastoid muscle
Internal jugular vein
External carotid artery

Parotid gland   Submandibular gland   Sublingual gland

FIGURE 7.24   SALIVARY GLAND STRUCTURE

The salivary glands serve several functions, including keeping the oral cavity moist and lubricated to protect it from abrasion, controlling oral bacteria by secreting lysozyme, liquefying the food (thereby allowing molecules within the food to interact with and stimulate the taste buds), secreting calcium and phosphate for tooth formation and maintenance, and secreting amylase to begin diges-tion of starches. The serous acinar cells secrete the protein and enzymatic components of saliva, whereas the mucous acinar cells secrete a watery (low-mucin) mucus. The parotid gland is com-posed entirely of serous acini. The sublingual gland contains pre-dominately mucous acini, with some serous acini as well. The sub-mandibular gland contains a mixture of serous and mucous acini.

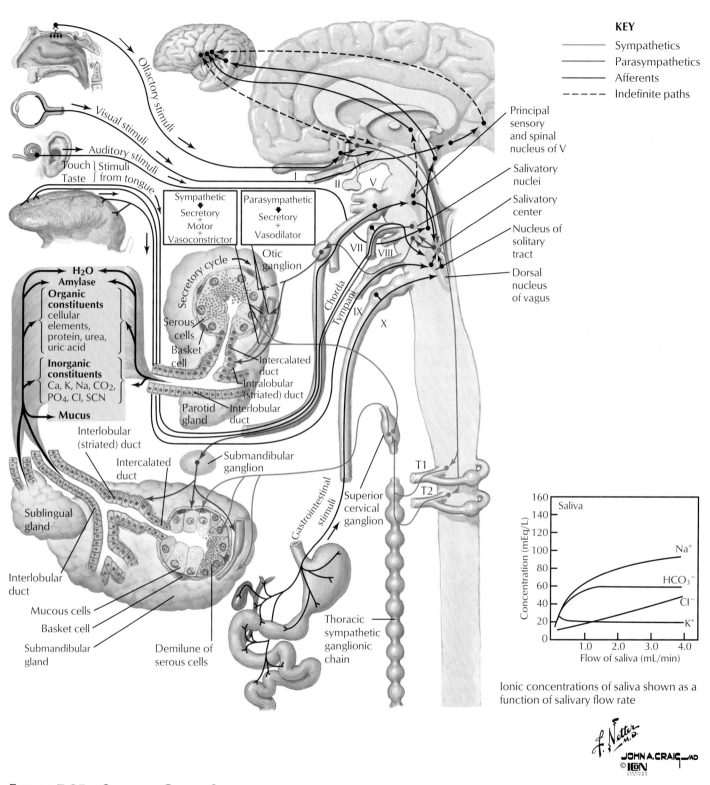

KEY

———	Sympathetics
———	Parasympathetics
———	Afferents
- - - -	Indefinite paths

Ionic concentrations of saliva shown as a function of salivary flow rate

FIGURE 7.25   SALIVARY GLAND SECRETION

The salivary gland is under autonomic control. The glands receive both sympathetic and parasympathetic input. Of these, the parasympathetic system is more important in stimulating secretion. The acinar cells secrete the protein (serous cells) and mucus (mucous cells) components of saliva. The acini also secrete a fluid component that has a composition similar to that of plasma. As the saliva makes its way out of the gland, the ductal cells modify its electrolyte composition by active transport, such that the saliva entering the mouth is hypotonic to plasma and has a high bicarbonate concentration.

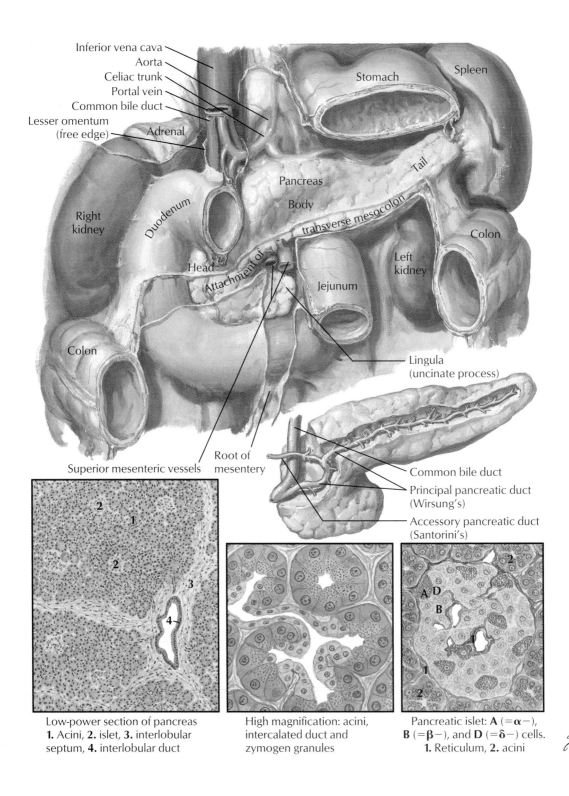

Low-power section of pancreas
1. Acini, **2.** islet, **3.** interlobular
septum, **4.** interlobular duct

High magnification: acini,
intercalated duct and
zymogen granules

Pancreatic islet: **A** ($=\alpha-$),
B ($=\beta-$), and **D** ($=\delta-$) cells.
1. Reticulum, **2.** acini

FIGURE 7.26 PANCREAS STRUCTURE

The pancreas has exocrine and endocrine components. The acinar cells of the exocrine pancreas secrete a number of enzymes that are necessary for digestion of protein, starches, and fats. The ductal cells secrete fluid, with a high HCO_3^- content. This HCO_3^- serves to neutralize the acid entering the duodenum from the stomach.

The endocrine pancreas consists of the islets of Langerhans. Within the islets, the A- or α-cells (located in the periphery of the islet) secrete glucagon, the B- or β-cells (located centrally in the islet) secrete insulin, and the D- or δ-cells (dispersed throughout the islet) secrete somatostatin.

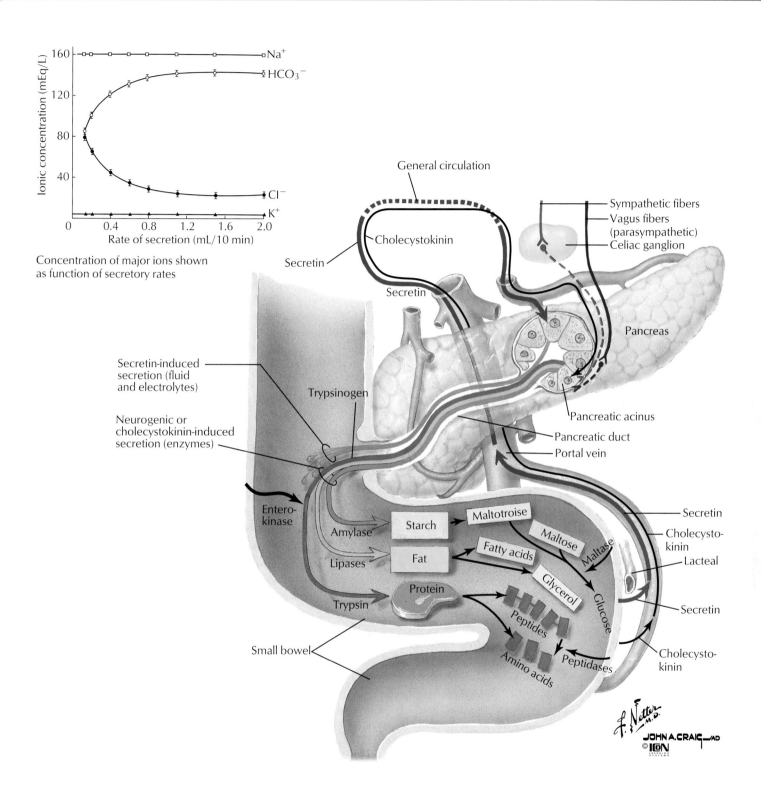

Concentration of major ions shown as function of secretory rates

FIGURE 7.27 PANCREAS SECRETION

Secretion by the pancreas in under neural and hormonal control. The parasympathetic system (vagus nerve) stimulates secretion. Secretin is secreted by the neuroendocrine S cells in response to the presence of acid in the duodenum. It acts on the ductal cells of the pancreas to stimulate the secretion of fluid with a high HCO_3^- content. Cholecystokinin is secreted by I cells in response to fats in the duodenum and upper jejunum. It acts on the acinar cells to stimulate the secretion of enzymes. *Not shown in the figure:* Trypsin in the lumen of the duodenum activates other protease precursors (chymotrypsinogen and procarboxypeptidase) to their active forms (chymotrypsin and carboxypeptidase). *Note:* Secretin and CCK are secreted throughout the duodenum, especially proximally.

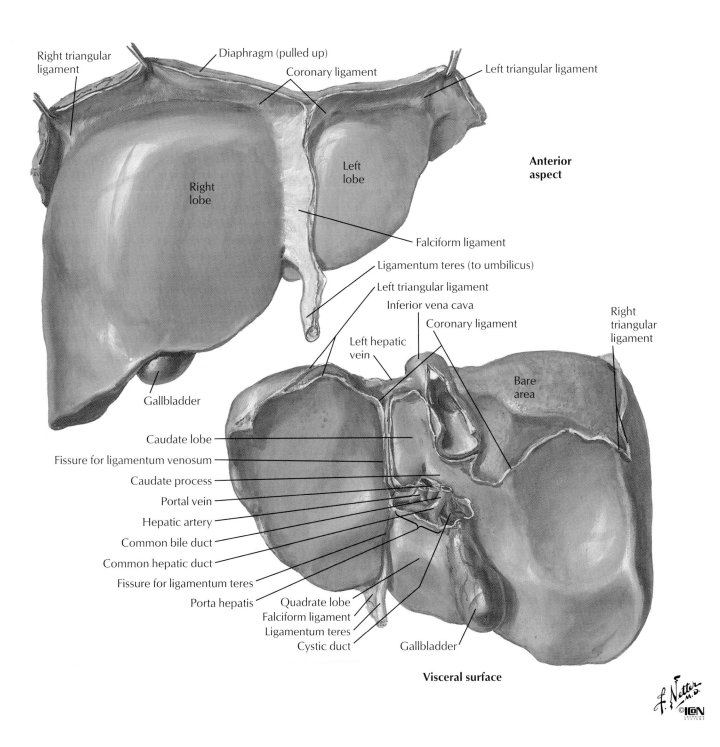

Right triangular ligament

Diaphragm (pulled up)

Coronary ligament

Left triangular ligament

Right lobe

Left lobe

Anterior aspect

Falciform ligament

Ligamentum teres (to umbilicus)

Left triangular ligament

Inferior vena cava

Coronary ligament

Right triangular ligament

Left hepatic vein

Bare area

Gallbladder

Caudate lobe

Fissure for ligamentum venosum

Caudate process

Portal vein

Hepatic artery

Common bile duct

Common hepatic duct

Fissure for ligamentum teres

Porta hepatis

Quadrate lobe

Falciform ligament

Ligamentum teres

Cystic duct

Gallbladder

Visceral surface

FIGURE 7.28 LIVER STRUCTURE

The liver is the largest gland in the body and consists of four anatomical lobes (right, left, quadrate, and caudate). Various ligaments attach the liver to the overlying diaphragm (coronary ligaments) and anterior abdominal wall (falciform ligament). Functionally, the liver has two lobes (right and left), and each lobe receives arterial blood from the hepatic artery and portal venous blood from the abdominal GI tract. Each lobe also possesses its own venous and biliary drainage.

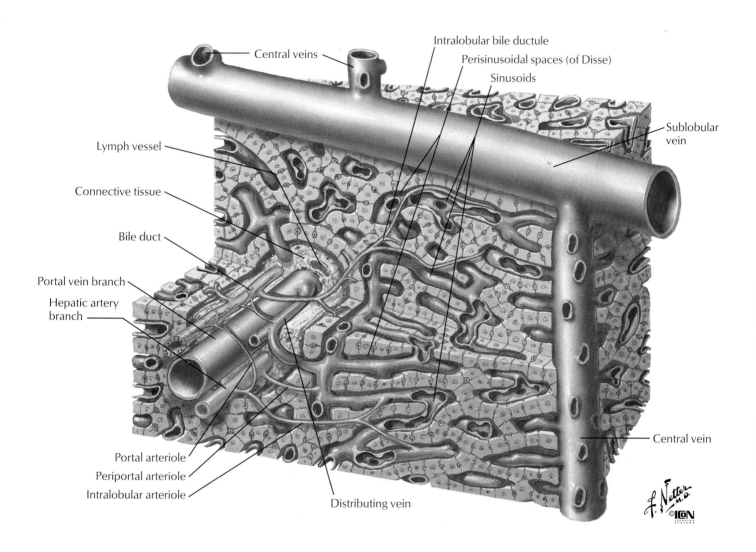

FIGURE 7.29   LIVER ULTRASTRUCTURE

The liver cells (hepatocytes) receive blood from the portal circulation (75%) and from the hepatic artery (25%). Hepatocytes are arranged in plates of cells that are separated from each other by hepatic sinusoids. The blood moves from the portal vein and hepatic arteriole branches through the sinusoids to the central vein. From the central vein, blood flows into the hepatic veins and inferior vena cava. The sinusoids are lined by a discontinuous endothelium that allows free movement of proteins from the blood to the hepatocytes, as well as from the hepatocytes to the blood. The sinusoids also contain phagocytic cells (Kupffer cells) that clear damaged red blood cells and foreign antigens (not shown). Bile is produced by the hepatocytes and drains into intralobular bile ductules and then larger bile ducts (right and left). The bile ducts coarse with the hepatic artery and portal vein. Ultimately, bile is collected into the gallbladder, where it is stored and concentrated.

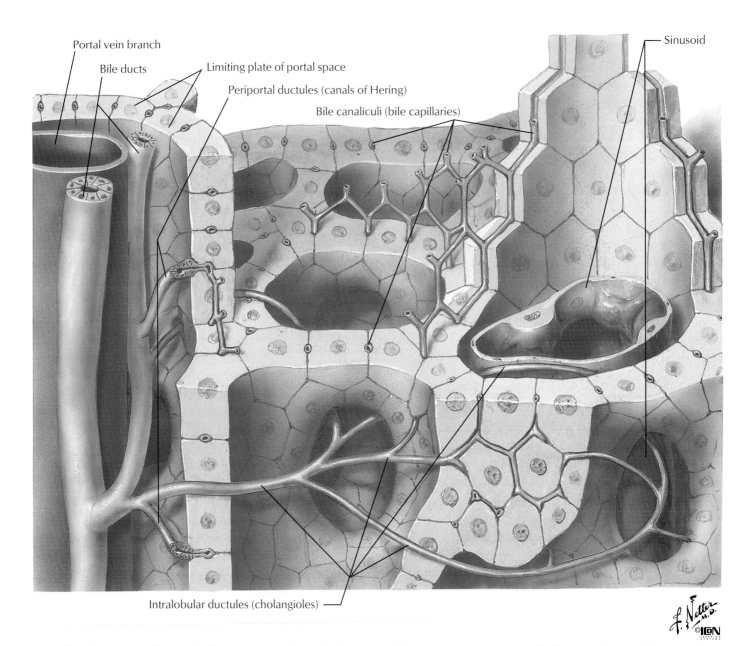

Note: The figure shows bile canaliculi as structures with walls of their own. However, boundaries of canaliculi are really a specialization of surface membranes of adjacent liver cells

FIGURE 7.30   INTRAHEPATIC BILIARY SYSTEM

The hepatocytes secrete bile into the bile canaliculi (approximately 500 mL/day of bile is produced). Bile flows from the canaliculi to the intralobular ductules and then empties into the bile ducts that run with the portal vein and hepatic artery branches.

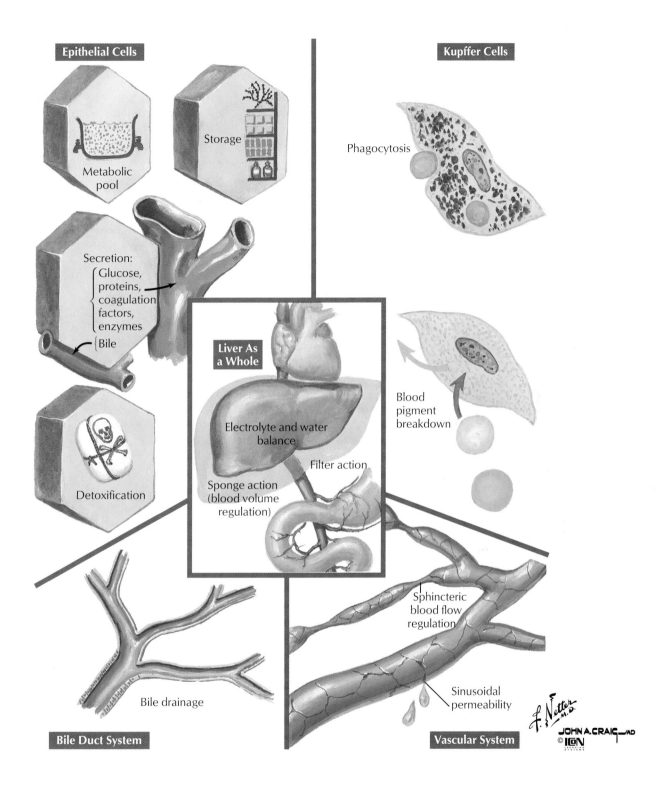

FIGURE 7.31 OVERVIEW OF LIVER FUNCTION

The liver serves a number of important functions, including storage of important products and energy sources (e.g., glycogen, fat, protein, and vitamins), production of cellular fuels (e.g., glucose, fatty acids, and keto acids), production of plasma proteins and clotting factors, metabolism of toxins and drugs, the excretion of substances (e.g., bilirubin), and the production of bile acids. The Kupf-fer cells phagocytose foreign materials that cross the wall of the GI tract and enter the portal circulation. Cells of the mononuclear phagocytic system (MPS), both in the liver (i.e., Kupffer cells) and throughout the body phagocytose damaged red blood cells. Bilirubin is a product of hemoglobin degradation, and it excreted by the liver in the bile (see Figure 7.32).

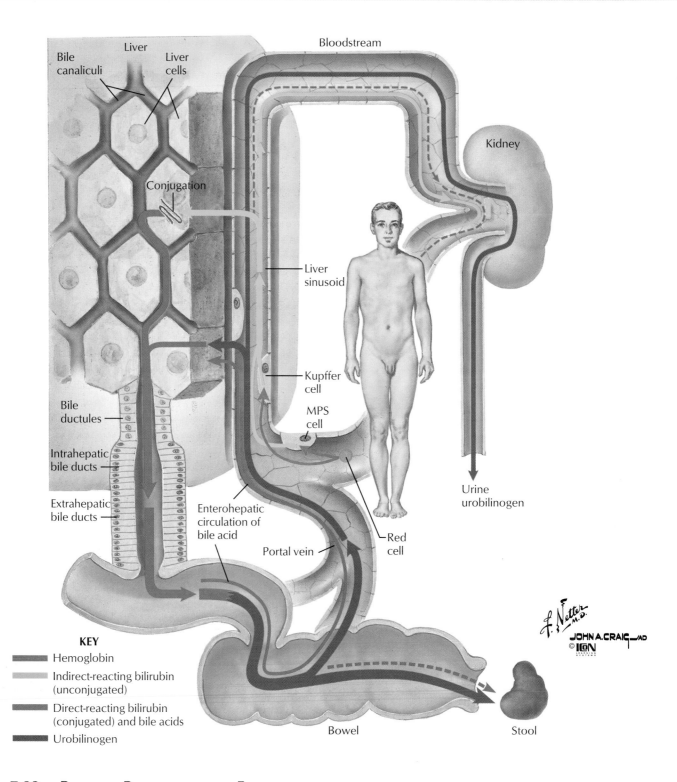

FIGURE 7.32 BILIRUBIN PRODUCTION AND EXCRETION

Cells of the mononuclear phagocytic system (MPS), both in the liver (i.e., Kupffer cells) and throughout the body, phagocytose damaged red blood cells. Bilirubin, a degradation product of hemoglobin, is produced by these cells (unconjugated bilirubin). The liver hepatocytes take up this bilirubin, conjugate it with glucuronic acid (conjugated bilirubin), and excrete it into the bile. In the intestine the bilirubin is converted to urobilinogen by bacterial action. Some of this urobilinogen is absorbed and returned to the liver, which reexcretes it in the bile. Some of the urobilinogen is also excreted by the kidneys. The bile also contains bile acids, which aid in the digestion of lipids by their ability to emulsify fats and form mixed micelles with the lipid molecules (see Figure 7.37). Bile acids are reabsorbed by the terminal ileum. Typically, 65% to 85% of the bile acids are recirculated in this manner (enterohepatic circulation). The bile acids lost in the feces each day are replaced by hepatic synthesis.

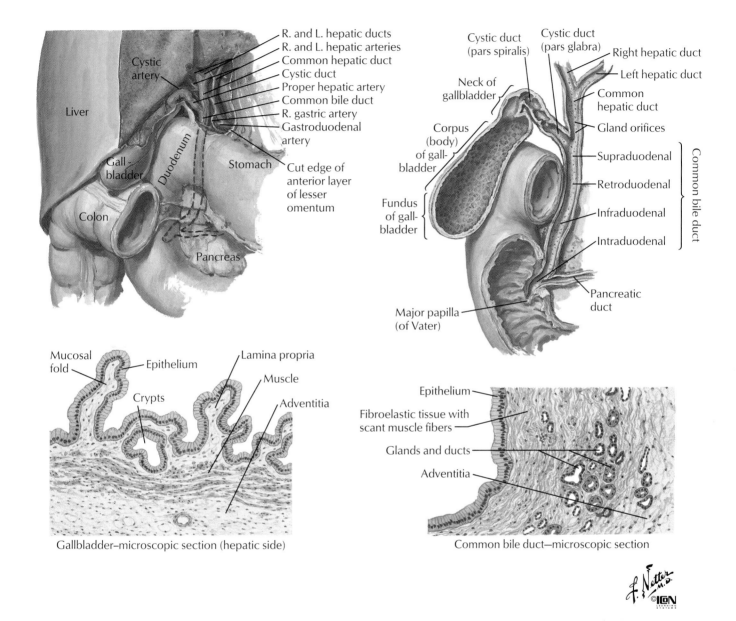

FIGURE 7.33 GALLBLADDER STRUCTURE AND FUNCTION

The gallbladder is a small hollow organ attached to the surface of the liver. It serves to store and concentrate the bile synthesized by the liver (holds about 20 to 50 mL of bile). Vagal stimulation and cholecystokinin released from neuroendocrine cells in the duodenum (in response to the presence of fat) cause the gallbladder to contract and transport bile down the cystic duct and the common bile duct, where it empties into the second (descending) portion of the duodenum. The gallbladder mucosa is specialized for electrolyte and water absorption, which allows the gallbladder to concentrate the bile.

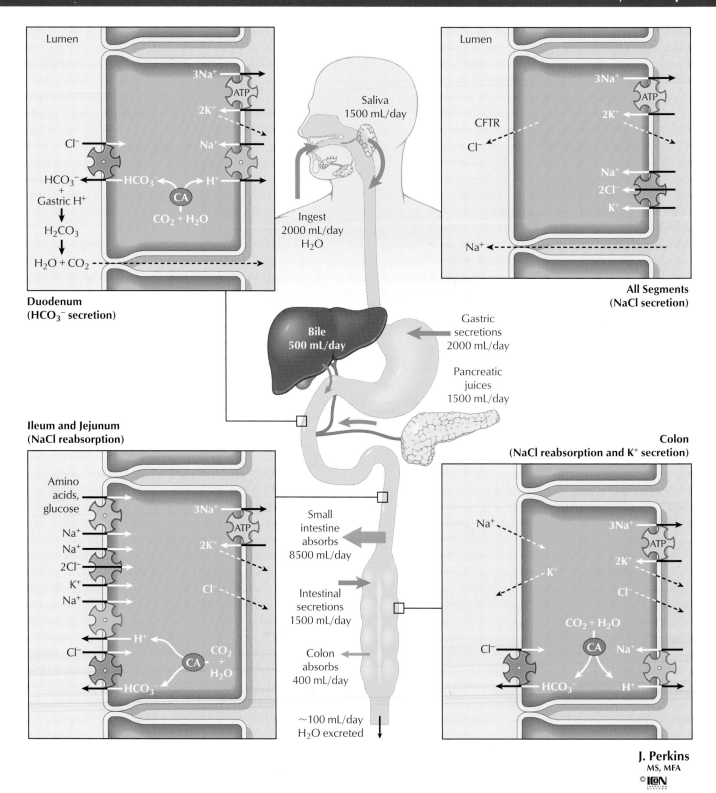

Duodenum (HCO₃⁻ secretion)

All Segments (NaCl secretion)

Ileum and Jejunum (NaCl reabsorption)

Colon (NaCl reabsorption and K⁺ secretion)

Saliva 1500 mL/day

Ingest 2000 mL/day H₂O

Bile 500 mL/day

Gastric secretions 2000 mL/day

Pancreatic juices 1500 mL/day

Small intestine absorbs 8500 mL/day

Intestinal secretions 1500 mL/day

Colon absorbs 400 mL/day

~100 mL/day H₂O excreted

J. Perkins
MS, MFA
© ICN

FIGURE 7.34   GI TRACT FLUID AND ELECTROLYTE TRANSPORT

Large volumes of fluid are secreted and absorbed by the GI tract each day. The secreted fluid helps maintain the intestinal contents in a liquefied state to aid digestion. Normally, this secreted fluid, along with any fluid ingested, is absorbed so that only 100 mL/day of water is excreted in the feces (with diarrhea, intestinal fluid loss can reach 20 L/day). Both the secretion of fluid and its absorption are driven by electrolyte transport. Secretion of NaCl drives fluid secretion, whereas the absorption of Na⁺ with Cl⁻ and other solutes drives absorption. The principal cellular mechanisms of intestinal electrolyte transport are illustrated. For simplicity, not all known mechanisms are shown. Also, cells may express multiple transport systems, which here are depicted as being present in different cells.

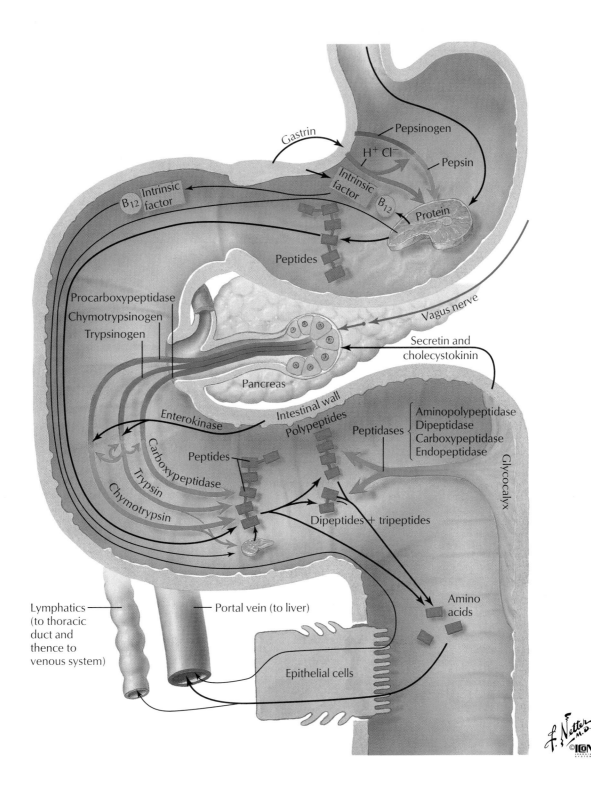

FIGURE 7.35   DIGESTION OF PROTEIN

Protein digestion begins in the stomach through the action of HCl and pepsin. Pancreatic proteases and peptidases associated with the glycocalyx of the intestinal epithelial cells continue this process, yielding amino acids, tripeptides, and dipeptides, which are then absorbed by the intestinal epithelial cells. The tripeptides and dipeptides are absorbed coupled to H^+, while the amino acids are absorbed coupled to Na^+ (see Figure 7.34).

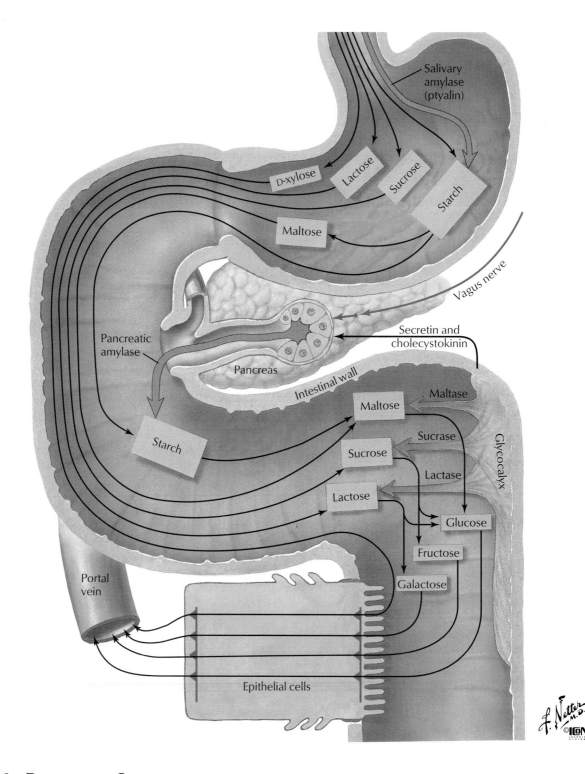

FIGURE 7.36 DIGESTION OF CARBOHYDRATES

Digestion of carbohydrates and starches begins in the mouth and stomach through the action of salivary amylase. Pancreatic amylase and enzymes associated with the glycocalyx of the intestinal epithelial cells continue this process, yielding monosaccharides. These monosaccharides are absorbed by the intestinal epithelial cells coupled to Na$^+$ (see Figure 7.34).

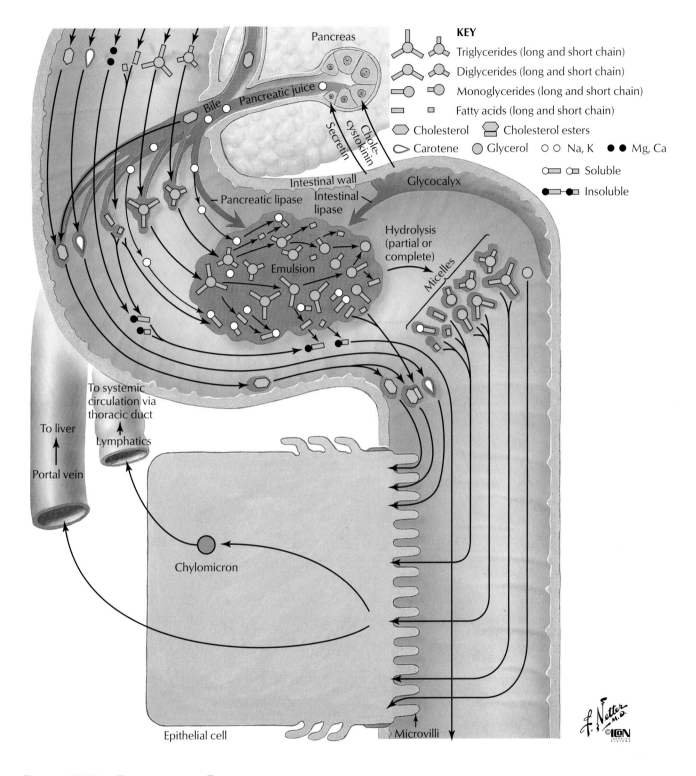

FIGURE 7.37   DIGESTION OF FAT

Fat digestion begins in the intestine, largely by the action of pancreatic lipases. Lipases associated with the glycocalyx of the epithelial cells also contribute to this process. The bile salts are critically important in this process because they emulsify the fats and form mixed micelles. Soluble glycerol and some smaller chained fatty acids are absorbed without micelle formation. The cellular mechanisms for absorption of the products of fat digestion are not completely known. The principal forms absorbed by the intestinal epithelial cells are fatty acids (absorbed coupled to Na$^+$),

monoglycerides, and cholesterol. Further processing within the epithelial cells results in chylomicron formation, and these chylomicrons are exocytosed at the basal membrane and taken up into lymphatic lacteals. They enter the thoracic duct and are eventually emptied into the venous system. Divalent cations in the lumen of the intestine can form insoluble complexes, preventing absorption. By this same mechanism, malabsorption of fat can impair intestinal Ca^{2+} absorption.

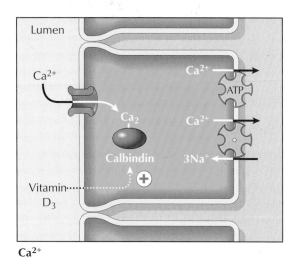

Ca²⁺

Iron

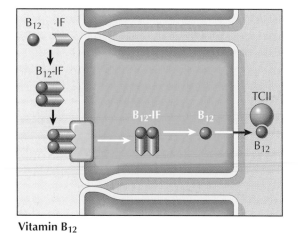

Water-Soluble Vitamins

Vitamin B₁₂

Fat-Soluble Vitamins

Element	Site of Absorption	Mechanism
Ca²⁺	Duodenum and jejunum	Active
Fe²⁺	Duodenum and jejunum	Facilitated diffusion
Water-Soluble Vitamins		
Vitamin C	Ileum	Na⁺-coupled/2° active
Thiamin (B₁)	Jejunum	Na⁺-coupled/2° active
Riboflavin (B₂)	Jejunum	Na⁺-coupled/2° active
Biotin	Jejunum	Na⁺-coupled/2° active
Vitamin B₁₂	Ileum	Facilitated diffusion
Pyridoxine (B₆)	Jejunum and ileum	Passive diffusion
Fat-Soluble Vitamins		
Vitamin A	Jejunum and ileum	Passive diffusion
Vitamin D	Jejunum and ileum	Passive diffusion
Vitamin E	Jejunum and ileum	Passive diffusion
Vitamin K	Jejunum and ileum	Passive diffusion

J. Perkins
MS, MFA
© ICON

FIGURE 7.38   ABSORPTION OF ESSENTIAL VITAMINS AND ELEMENTS

The cell mechanisms involved in the absorption of Ca²⁺, iron, and several important vitamins are summarized. Vitamin D₃ (1,25-dihydroxy-vitamin D₃) plays an important role in stimulating intestinal Ca²⁺ absorption. Intrinsic factor is made by the stomach (see Figure 7.12). If insufficient amounts of intrinsic factor are produced, B₁₂ deficiency ensues. Failure to properly digest fats (see Figure 7.37) can lead to deficiencies of the fat-soluble vitamins. *Abbreviations: DMT1*, Divalent metal transporter 1; *H*, hephaestin; *IF*, intrinsic factor; *IREG1*, iron-regulated transporter 1; *TCII*, transcobalamin II; *TF*, transferrin.

Chapter 8 Endocrine Physiology

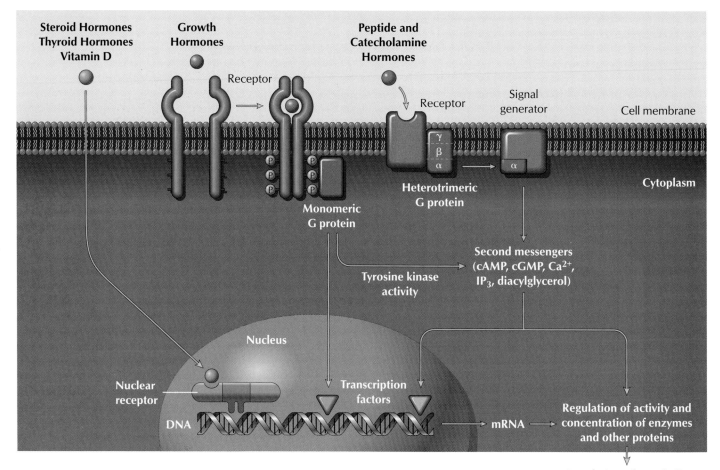

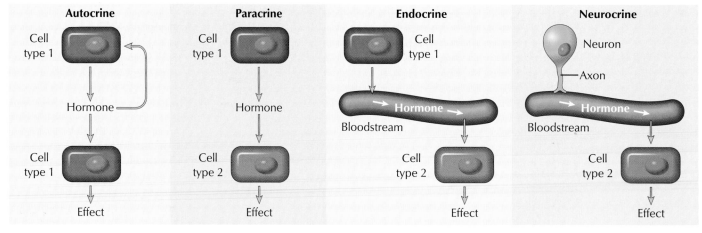

FIGURE 8.1   OVERVIEW OF HORMONE ACTION

Hormones are involved in the process of cell-to-cell signaling. Hormones interact with their target cells via specific hormone-receptor interactions (see Chart 1.2). The receptor may be in the plasma membrane or inside the cell (cytoplasmic or nuclear). The hormone-receptor interaction may generate second messengers or regulate gene expression. The effect of the hormone on the cell may be the result of altered metabolic pathways (i.e., changes in enzyme activity or concentrations of enzymes) or changes in cell structure and growth. The lower panel illustrates the different modes of cell-to-cell communication.

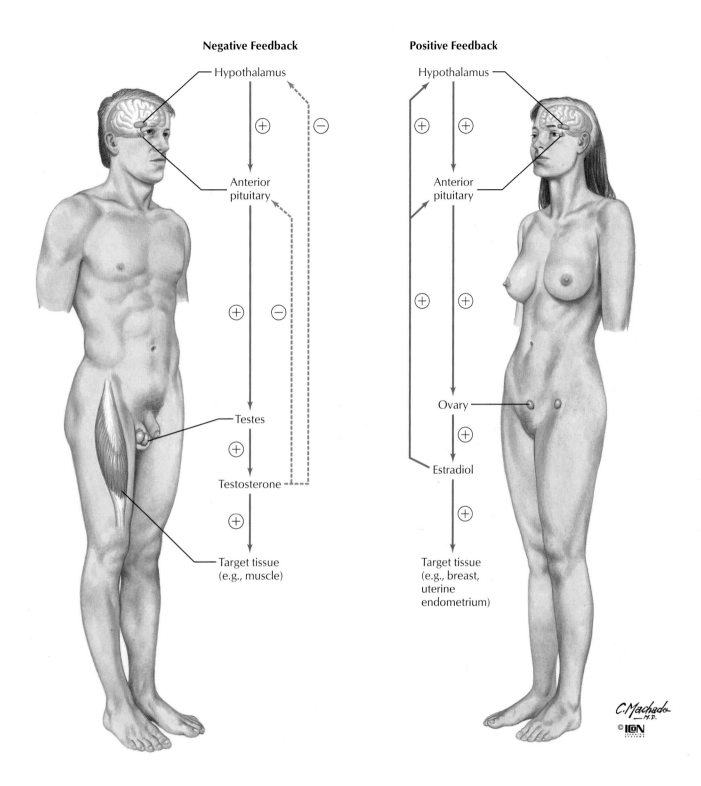

FIGURE 8.2 FEEDBACK REGULATION

Hormone secretion is regulated by both negative feedback mechanisms (e.g., testosterone) and positive feedback mechanisms (e.g., follicular phase of the menstrual cycle).

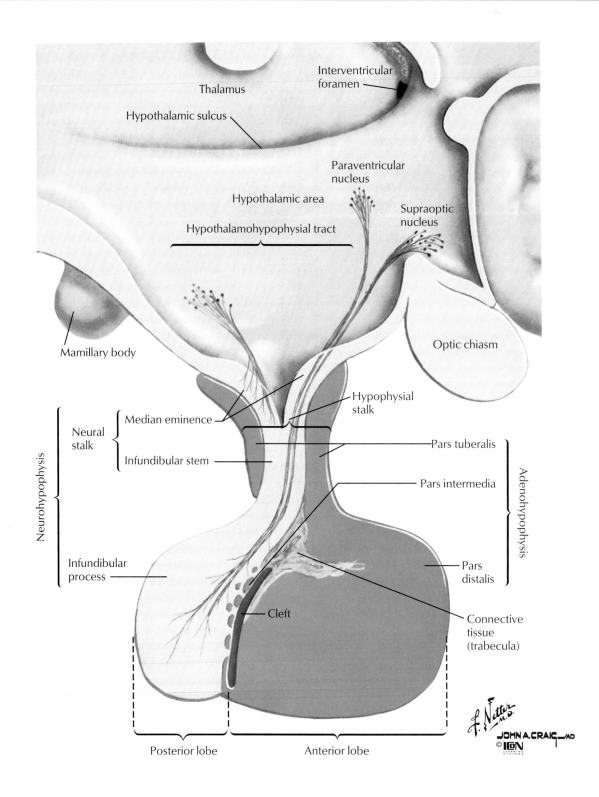

FIGURE 8.3 STRUCTURE OF HYPOTHALAMUS AND PITUITARY

The neurohypophysis (posterior pituitary) is formed as a downgrowth of the diencephalon of the brain. The adenohypophysis (anterior pituitary) is derived from Rathke's pouch (ectodermal tissue in the oropharynx). The intermediate lobe is not well developed in humans. Neuroendocrine cells in the hypothalamus send axons into the posterior pituitary and to the region of the median eminence. Hormones are released from these axons into the systemic blood (posterior pituitary) or into the hypothalamic-hypophyseal portal system (see Figure 8.4) in the region of the median eminence.

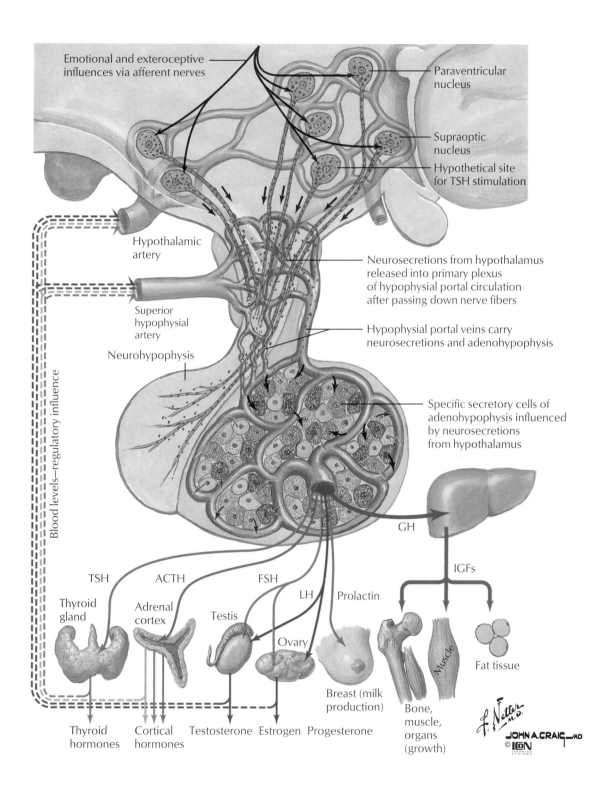

FIGURE 8.4   OVERVIEW OF ANTERIOR PITUITARY FUNCTION

Hypothalamic neuroendocrine cells release hormones into the hypothalamic-hypophyseal portal system that stimulate or inhibit the secretory cells of the anterior pituitary. Under the control of these hypothalamic releasing and inhibiting hormones, the cells of the anterior pituitary release tropic hormones, which then act on endocrine glands. The hormones secreted by the endocrine glands feedback on both the cells of the anterior pituitary and the hypothalamus to regulate the secretion of tropic hormones and releasing hormones.

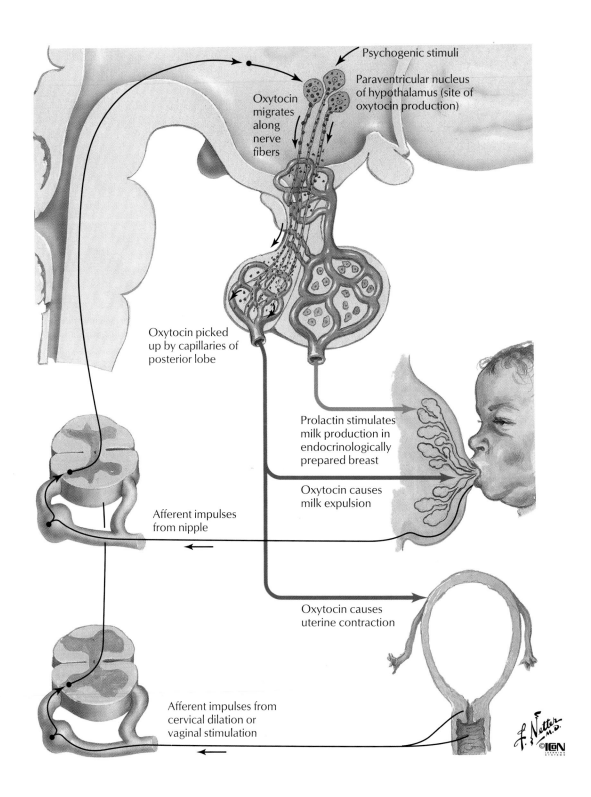

Psychogenic stimuli

Paraventricular nucleus of hypothalamus (site of oxytocin production)

Oxytocin migrates along nerve fibers

Oxytocin picked up by capillaries of posterior lobe

Prolactin stimulates milk production in endocrinologically prepared breast

Oxytocin causes milk expulsion

Afferent impulses from nipple

Oxytocin causes uterine contraction

Afferent impulses from cervical dilation or vaginal stimulation

Figure 8.5 Posterior Pituitary Function (Oxytocin)

Oxytocin is released from the posterior pituitary in response to vaginal stimulation and suckling. In response to vaginal stimulation, as occurs during sexual intercourse, oxytocin is released and causes uterine contraction. This may facilitate sperm transport through the uterus and uterine tubes. Oxytocin also facilitates childbirth by increasing uterine contractions during labor. During nursing, stimulation of the nipple by the suckling infant causes oxytocin release, which then acts on the myoepithelial cells surrounding the mammary gland alveoli and ducts causing expression of milk. Neural pathways activated during suckling also stimulate the secretion of prolactin.

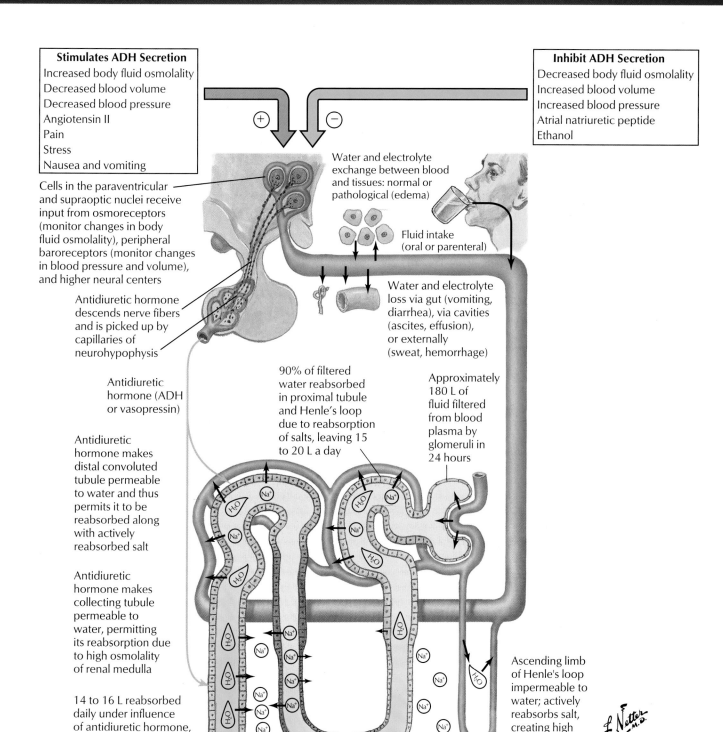

Stimulates ADH Secretion
Increased body fluid osmolality
Decreased blood volume
Decreased blood pressure
Angiotensin II
Pain
Stress
Nausea and vomiting

Inhibit ADH Secretion
Decreased body fluid osmolality
Increased blood volume
Increased blood pressure
Atrial natriuretic peptide
Ethanol

Cells in the paraventricular and supraoptic nuclei receive input from osmoreceptors (monitor changes in body fluid osmolality), peripheral baroreceptors (monitor changes in blood pressure and volume), and higher neural centers

Antidiuretic hormone descends nerve fibers and is picked up by capillaries of neurohypophysis

Antidiuretic hormone (ADH or vasopressin)

Antidiuretic hormone makes distal convoluted tubule permeable to water and thus permits it to be reabsorbed along with actively reabsorbed salt

Antidiuretic hormone makes collecting tubule permeable to water, permitting its reabsorption due to high osmolality of renal medulla

14 to 16 L reabsorbed daily under influence of antidiuretic hormone, resulting in 1 to 2 L of urine in 24 hours

Water and electrolyte exchange between blood and tissues: normal or pathological (edema)

Fluid intake (oral or parenteral)

Water and electrolyte loss via gut (vomiting, diarrhea), via cavities (ascites, effusion), or externally (sweat, hemorrhage)

90% of filtered water reabsorbed in proximal tubule and Henle's loop due to reabsorption of salts, leaving 15 to 20 L a day

Approximately 180 L of fluid filtered from blood plasma by glomeruli in 24 hours

Ascending limb of Henle's loop impermeable to water; actively reabsorbs salt, creating high osmolality of renal medulla

FIGURE 8.6 POSTERIOR PITUITARY FUNCTION (ADH)

Antidiuretic hormone (ADH), or vasopressin, is involved in the regulation of water balance. Changes in body fluid osmolality and blood volume and pressure are the primary physiologic regulators of ADH secretion (see also Figure 6.9). When ADH levels are elevated, a small volume of concentrated urine is excreted. When ADH levels are low, a large volume of dilute urine is excreted.

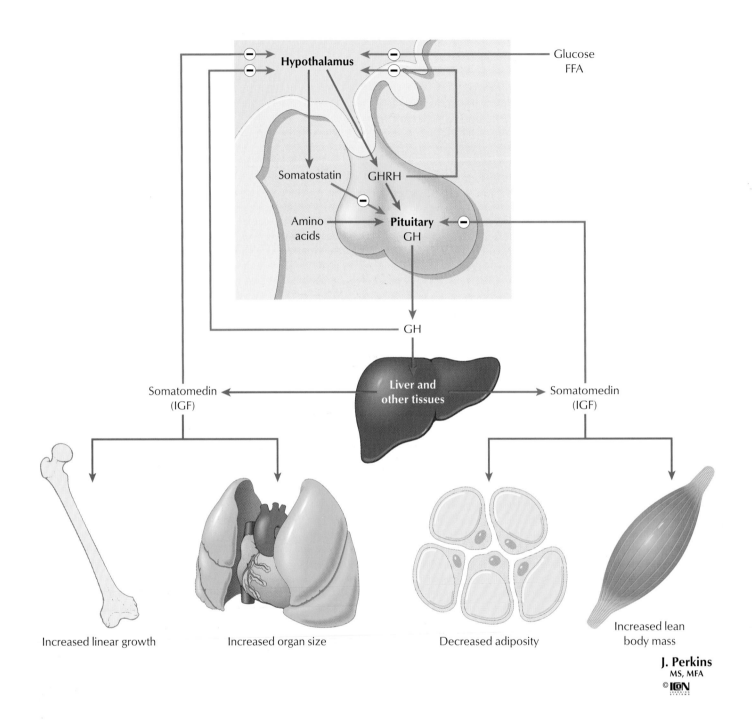

FIGURE 8.7   GROWTH HORMONE

Growth hormone's major physiological effect is to stimulate growth and development in children and adolescents. It also plays an important role in regulating overall body metabolism. Growth hormone produces many of effects through the generation, and then subsequent action of somatomedins such as insulin-like growth factor (IGF). *Abbreviations: FFA,* Free fatty acids; *GHRH,* growth hormone–releasing hormone.

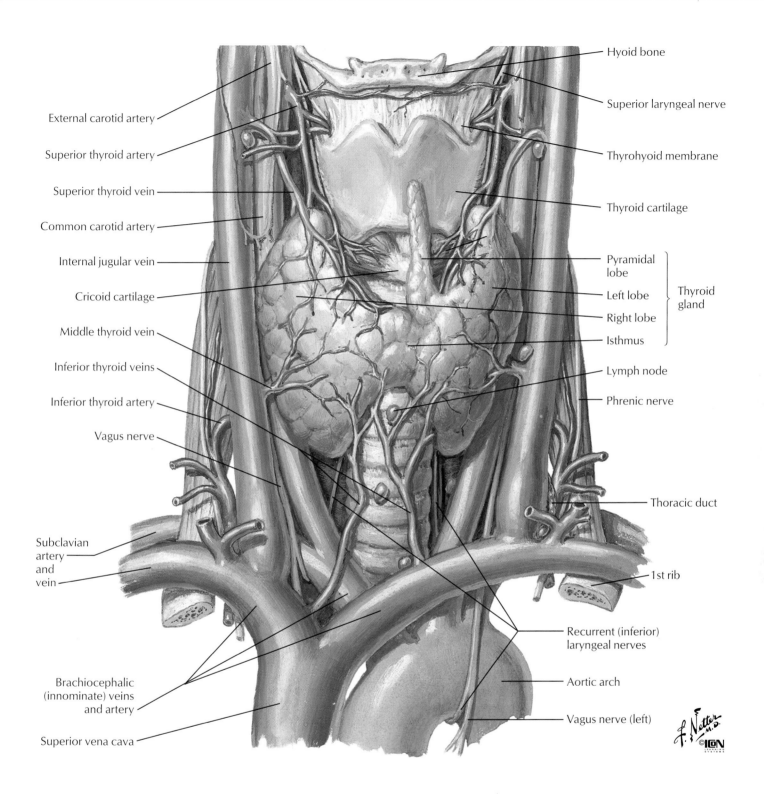

External carotid artery

Superior thyroid artery

Superior thyroid vein

Common carotid artery

Internal jugular vein

Cricoid cartilage

Middle thyroid vein

Inferior thyroid veins

Inferior thyroid artery

Vagus nerve

Subclavian artery and vein

Brachiocephalic (innominate) veins and artery

Superior vena cava

Hyoid bone

Superior laryngeal nerve

Thyrohyoid membrane

Thyroid cartilage

Pyramidal lobe

Left lobe

Right lobe

Isthmus

} Thyroid gland

Lymph node

Phrenic nerve

Thoracic duct

1st rib

Recurrent (inferior) laryngeal nerves

Aortic arch

Vagus nerve (left)

FIGURE 8.8 THYROID GLAND STRUCTURE

The thyroid gland is a ductless endocrine gland that weighs about 20 grams and consists of a right and left lobe joined by an isthmus. In 15% of the population, there is a small pyramidal lobe extend-ing cranially, as in this figure. The gland lies anterior to the trachea and just inferior to the cricoid cartilage. As with all endocrine glands, the thyroid has a rich vascular supply and venous drainage.

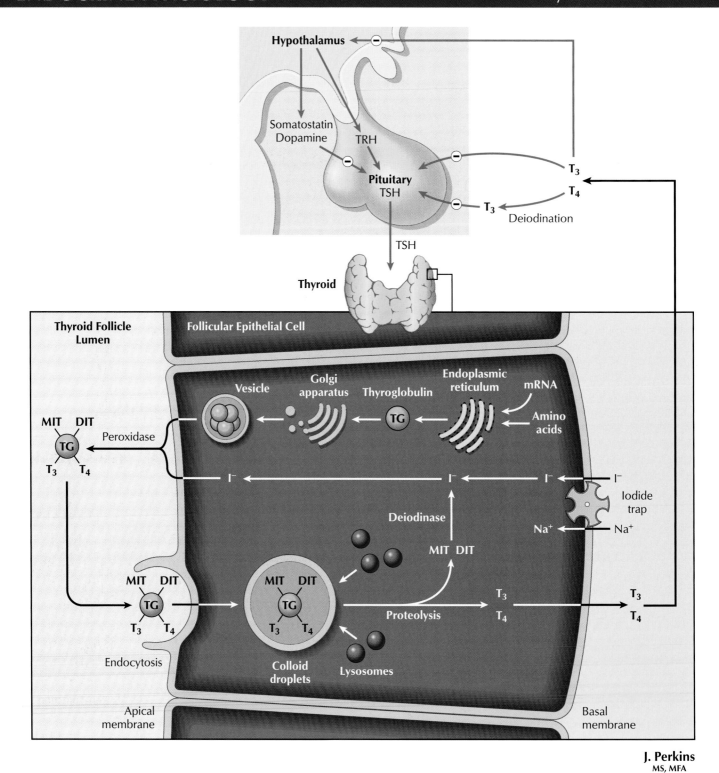

FIGURE 8.9 THYROID GLAND FUNCTION

The thyroid gland is composed of follicles formed by epithelial cells. These follicular epithelial cells synthesize, store, and secrete thyroxine (T_4) and triiodothyronine (T_3). The thyroid gland actively takes up iodide, iodinates tyrosine molecules (MIT = monoiodotyrosine; DIT = diiodotyrosine), couples these together to form T_4 and T_3, and stores these linked to thyroglobulin in the thyroid folli- cle. In the presence of thyroid-stimulating hormone (TSH), thy- roglobulin is endocytosed and T_3 and T_4 are released into the blood (TSH also stimulates the synthesis of T_3, T_4, and thyroglobulin). Most of the secreted hormone (90%) is in the form of T_4, which serves as a prehormone, because T_4 is converted to the more active form T_3 by peripheral tissues.

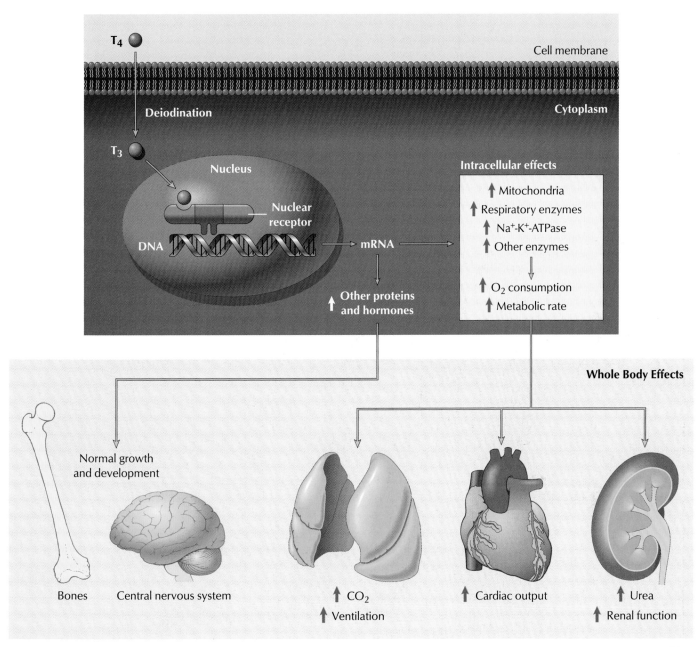

J. Perkins
MS, MFA
© ICN
LEARNING SYSTEMS

FIGURE 8.10   THYROID HORMONE ACTION

Thyroxine (T_4) is converted to triiodothyronine (T_3) at target tissues. T_3 binds to a nuclear receptor, resulting in transcription of a host of cellular proteins and enzymes. The net effect is an increase in metabolic rate and O_2 consumption. These effects are associated with increased heart, lung, and kidney function. T_3 is also important for normal growth and development.

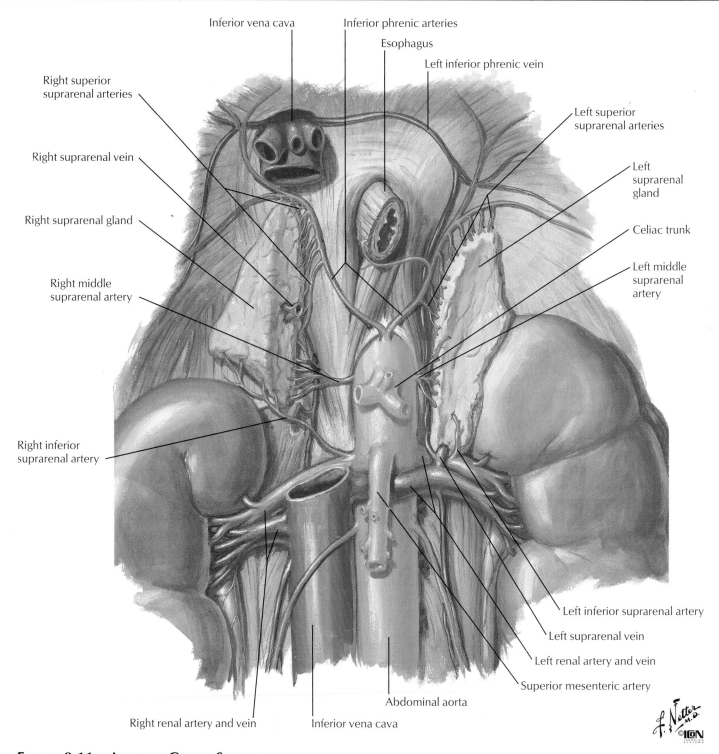

FIGURE 8.11 ADRENAL GLAND STRUCTURE

The paired adrenal (suprarenal) glands are retroperitoneal ductless endocrine glands that are nestled above the superior pole of each kidney and the overlying diaphragm. Each gland normally weighs about 7 to 8 grams, is highly vascularized, and consists of an outer cortex and an inner medulla (see Figure 8.12).

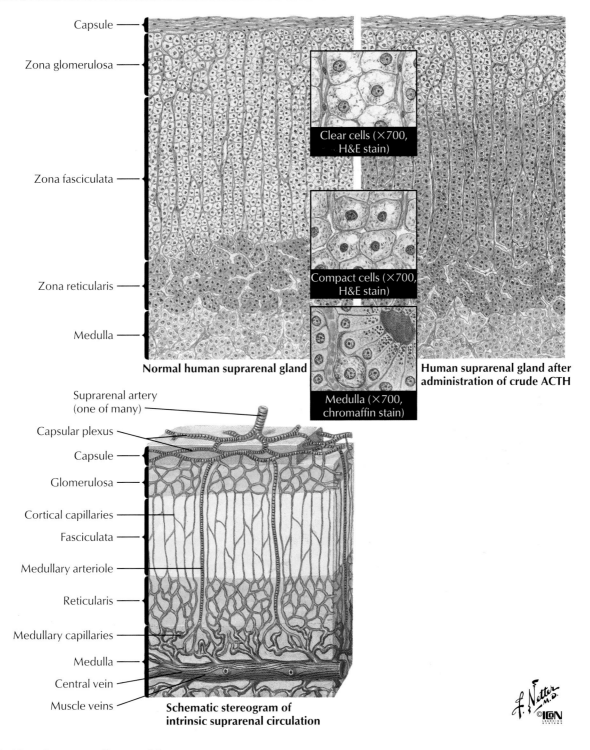

Capsule

Zona glomerulosa

Clear cells (×700, H&E stain)

Zona fasciculata

Zona reticularis

Compact cells (×700, H&E stain)

Medulla

Medulla (×700, chromaffin stain)

Normal human suprarenal gland

Human suprarenal gland after administration of crude ACTH

Suprarenal artery (one of many)

Capsular plexus

Capsule

Glomerulosa

Cortical capillaries

Fasciculata

Medullary arteriole

Reticularis

Medullary capillaries

Medulla

Central vein

Muscle veins

Schematic stereogram of intrinsic suprarenal circulation

FIGURE 8.12   ADRENAL GLAND HISTOLOGY

The adrenal gland consists of a cortex and medulla, and both regions are richly vascularized by a radially oriented plexus of vessels. The adrenal cortex produces more than two dozen steroid hormones and structurally is divided into three distinct histological regions: an outer zona glomerulosa that produces mineralocorticoids (principally aldosterone), a middle zona fasciculata that produces glucocorticoids (primarily cortisol, corticosterone, and cortisone), and an inner zona reticularis that produces androgens. As shown in this figure, ACTH stimulation significantly affects the maintenance and function of the inner two layers of the adrenal cortex. The adrenal medulla occupies the center of the adrenal gland and produces epinephrine and norepinephrine. The medullary cells actually are the postganglionic elements of the sympathetic division of the autonomic nervous system, but as endocrine cells, they release epinephrine and norepinephrine into the blood rather than into a synaptic cleft. Epinephrine accounts for about 70% to 80% of the medullary secretions. As illustrated in the lower panel, blood drains from the cortex into the medulla. This vascular arrangement ensures that the medulla receives large amounts of cortisol, which stimulates the enzyme that converts norepinephrine to epinephrine (i.e., phenylethanolamine-N-methyltransferase).

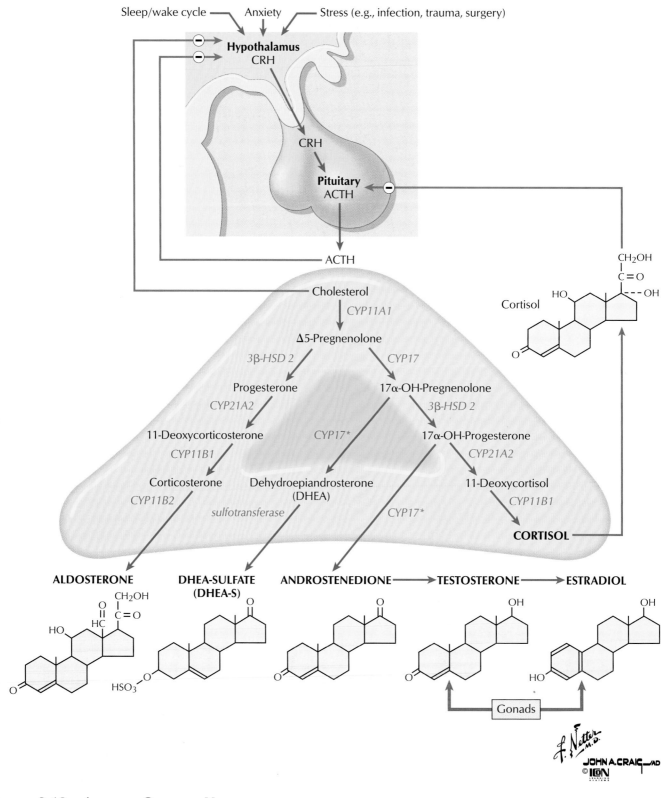

FIGURE 8.13   ADRENAL CORTICAL HORMONES

The adrenal cortex synthesizes and secretes glucocorticoid hormones (e.g., cortisol), mineralocorticoid hormones (e.g., aldosterone), and androgens (e.g., DHEA, androstenedione). Small amounts of circulating testosterone and estradiol are derived from the adrenal cortex, but the gonads are their primary source. All of the adrenal steroid hormones are derived from cholesterol. Cortisol secretion is under the control of adrenocorticotropic hormone (ACTH), which is secreted from the anterior pituitary in response to corticotropin-releasing hormone. ACTH also stimulates the production of adrenal androgens. ACTH is not the primary regulator of aldosterone secretion (see Figure 8.16). *Abbreviations: CYP11A1,* Side-chain cleavage; *3β-HSD 2,* 3β-hydroxysteroid dehydrogenase; *CYP21A2,* 21-hydroxylase; *CYP11B1,* 11β-hydroxylase; *CYP11B2,* aldosterone synthetase; *CYP17,* 17α-hydroxylase; *CTP17*,* 17,20-lyase.

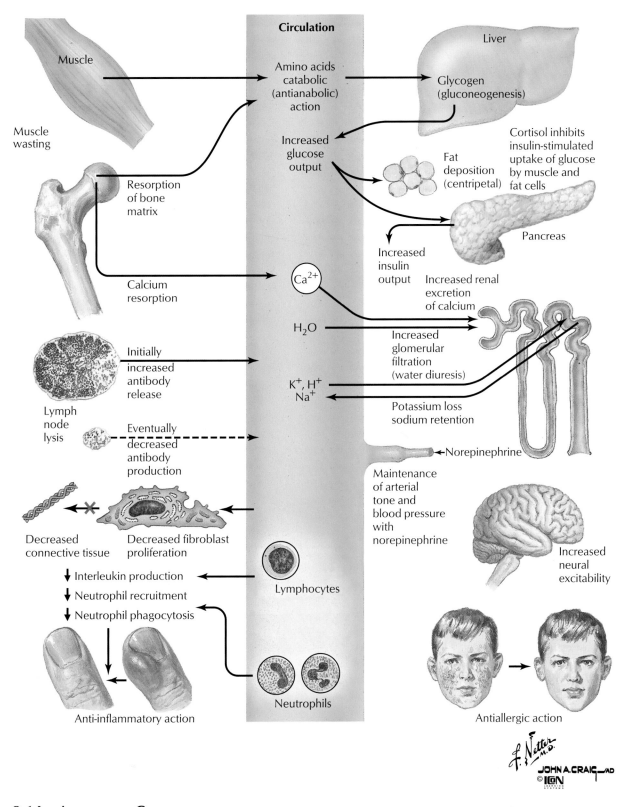

FIGURE 8.14   ACTIONS OF CORTISOL

Cortisol has many direct and indirect actions. It causes muscle wasting, fat deposition, hyperglycemia, insulin resistance, osteoporosis, suppression of the immune response (anti-inflammatory), and reduced production of connective tissue that can lead to poor wound healing. At high levels, it can exhibit mineralocorticoid actions and cause Na^+ retention and enhanced K^+ and H^+ excretion by the kidneys. Cortisol is also necessary for the normal production of epinephrine by the adrenal medulla (see Figure 8.17).

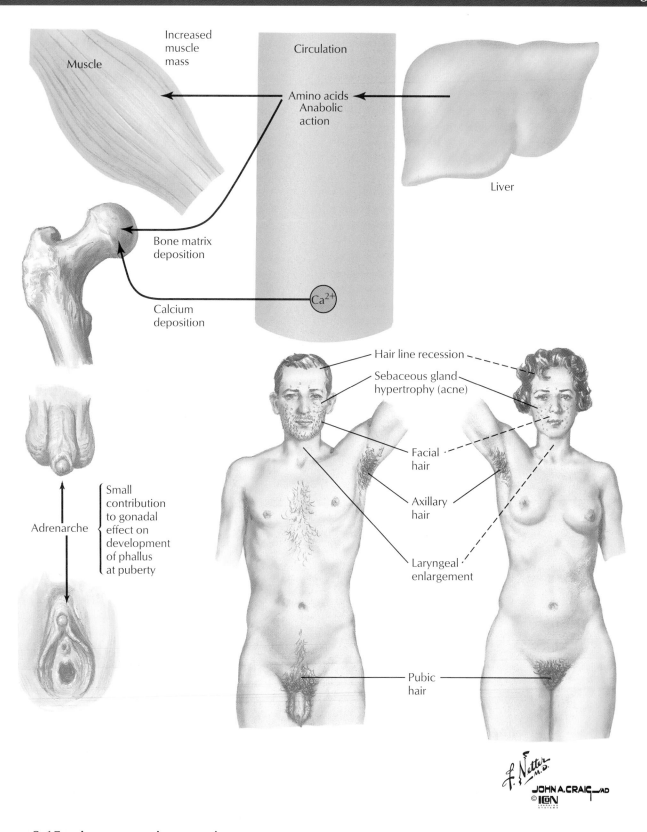

FIGURE 8.15   ACTIONS OF ADRENAL ANDROGENS

The adrenal androgens, dehydroepiandrosterone (DHEA) and androstenedione, do not have major effects in males, where the actions of testosterone predominate. In females, the adrenal glands are the primary source of circulating androgens. These adrenal androgens are responsible for the growth of both pubic and axillary hair. In both sexes, adrenal androgens play an important role in puberty. In early puberty, the adrenal androgens contribute to development of the external genitalia and other secondary sexual characteristics—a process termed adrenarche (see Figure 8.25). The general effects of androgens are anabolic, leading to increased muscle mass and bone formation. They also cause sebaceous gland hypertrophy, hairline recession, and growth of facial hair.

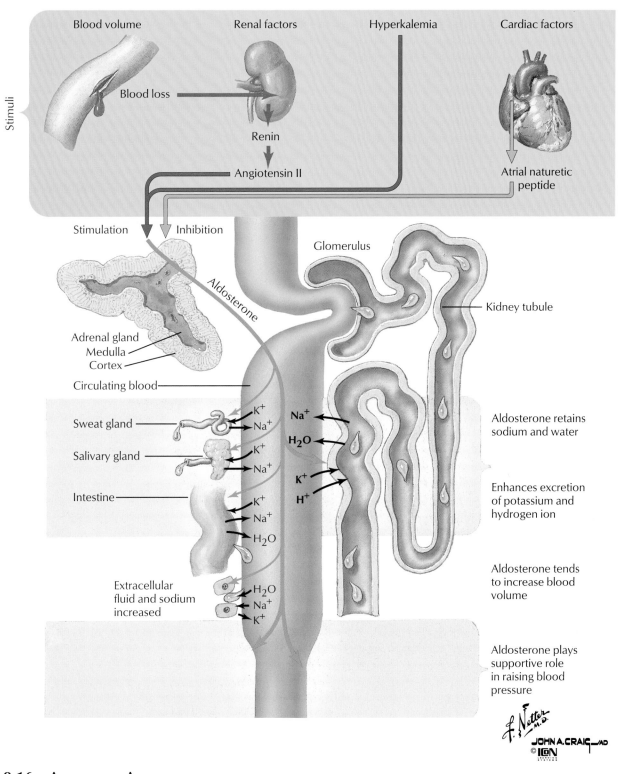

FIGURE 8.16 ACTIONS OF ALDOSTERONE

The mineralocorticoid aldosterone plays an important role in regulating the extracellular fluid (ECF) and blood volumes and in maintaining K^+ balance. When ECF and blood volumes are reduced (e.g., hemorrhage, diarrhea), renin is released from the kidney, which in turn increases angiotensin II levels. Angiotensin II is a potent stimulator of aldosterone secretion by the adrenal gland. Aldosterone acts on a number of organs, causing the retention of Na^+ and water, a response that serves to increase ECF and blood volume. The kidney is the most important organ in this response (see Figures 6.12 and 6.14). When the ECF and blood volumes are increased (e.g., congestive heart failure), atrial natriuretic peptide is secreted and acts on the adrenal cortex to inhibit aldosterone secretion (see Figure 6.13). An increase in the $[K^+]$ of the ECF (hyperkalemia) also stimulates aldosterone secretion by the adrenal cortex. Aldosterone acts primarily on the kidney to stimulate K^+ excretion (see Figure 6.15). Finally, aldosterone increases urinary H^+ excretion (see Figure 6.17).

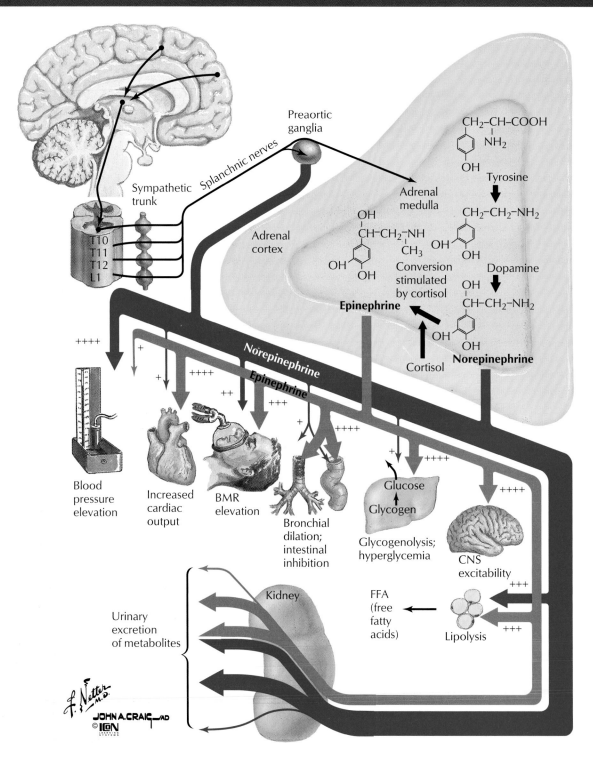

FIGURE 8.17   FUNCTION OF THE ADRENAL MEDULLA

The adrenal medulla produces epinephrine and norepinephrine. The medullary cells actually are the postganglionic elements of the sympathetic division of the autonomic nervous system, but as endocrine cells, they release epinephrine and norepinephrine into the blood rather than into a synaptic cleft. Epinephrine accounts for about 70% to 80% of the medullary secretions. The relative magnitude and effects of epinephrine and norepinephrine are illustrated.

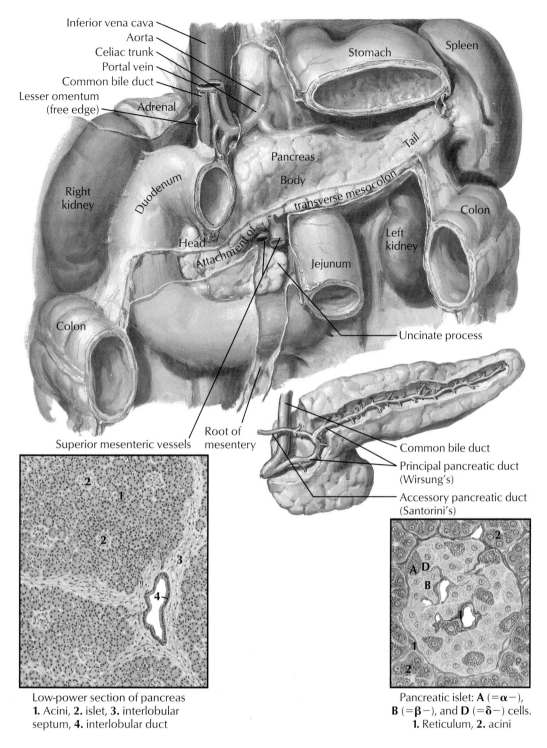

Low-power section of pancreas
1. Acini, 2. islet, 3. interlobular
septum, 4. interlobular duct

Pancreatic islet: **A** (=**α**−),
B (=**β**−), and **D** (=**δ**−) cells.
1. Reticulum, 2. acini

FIGURE 8.18   STRUCTURE OF THE ENDOCRINE PANCREAS

The pancreas is both an exocrine and endocrine gland. Its digestive enzymes are secreted into the duodenum via the pancreatic duct system, and about 99% of the cells are exocrine in function (see Figures 7.26 and 7.27). The endocrine portion of the pancreas is represented by clusters of islet cells (of Langerhans) (lower left micrograph), a heterogenous population of cells responsible for the elaboration and secretion of glucagon (α-cells), insulin (β-cells), and somatostatin (δ-cells). Glucagon is a fuel-mobilization hor-mone (see Figure 8.21). Insulin is a fuel-storage hormone (see Figure 8.20). Somatostatin has a number of actions in the GI tract; within the islets, it acts on both the α- and β-cells to suppress glucagon and insulin secretion. A fourth cell type, the F cell (not shown), secretes pancreatic polypeptide whose primary action is to inhibit the secretion of enzymes and HCO_3^- by the exocrine component of the pancreas.

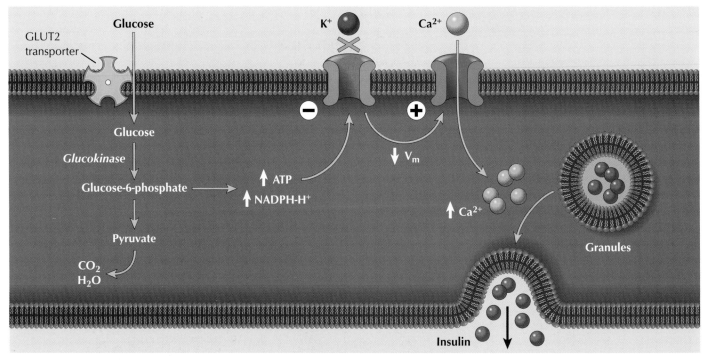

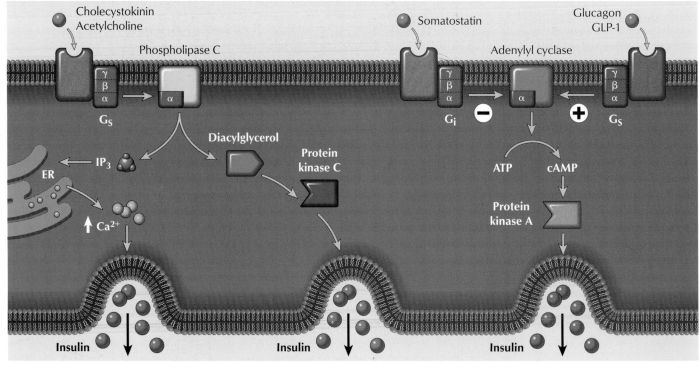

J. Perkins
MS, MFA
©ICN

FIGURE 8.19   INSULIN SECRETION

The most important factor regulating insulin secretion is the glucose concentration of the blood. When the blood glucose concentration increases, insulin secretion is stimulated. Glucose enters the cell, where its metabolism increases intracellular ATP levels. The increased ATP levels close an ATP-dependent K^+ channel in the plasma membrane and thereby depolarize the membrane potential (V_m). This membrane potential depolarization opens voltage-sensitive Ca^{2+} channels, and the intracellular $[Ca^{2+}]$ increases. The rise in intracellu-

lar $[Ca^{2+}]$ triggers exocytosis of the insulin-containing secretory granules. Other factors potentiate this effect of glucose on insulin secretion. Hormones and candidate hormones released by neuroendocrine cells in the intestine during digestion facilitate insulin secretion. These hormones and candidate hormones include cholecystokinin, glucagon-like peptide (GLP-1) and glucagon. Acetylcholine (from vagal efferents) also stimulates insulin secretion, while somatostatin from the islet δ-cells inhibits secretion.

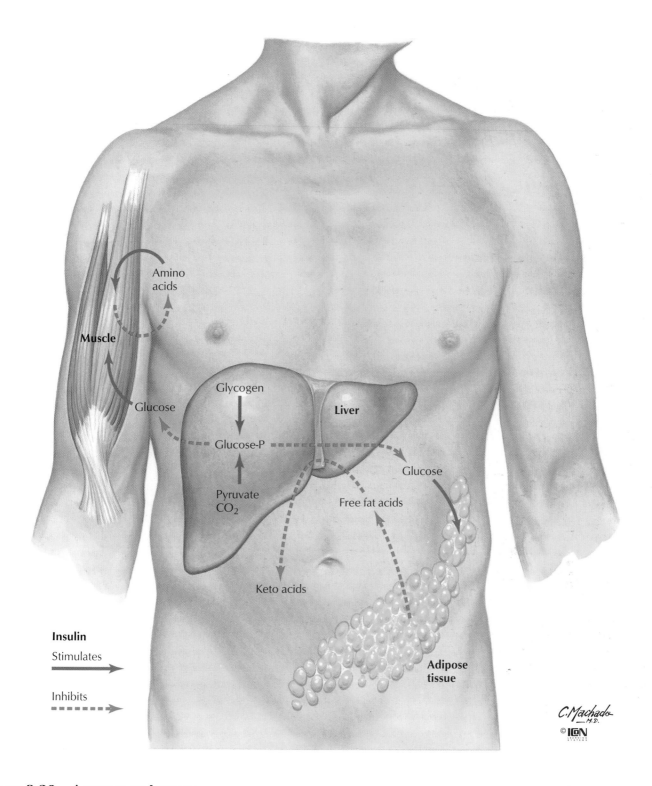

FIGURE 8.20 ACTIONS OF INSULIN

Insulin is a fuel-storage hormone. The major fuels used by cells are glucose, fatty acids, and keto acids (derived during fatty acid metabolism). Some cells preferentially use glucose as their fuel (e.g., neurons), whereas other cells preferentially use fatty acids (e.g., skeletal muscle). Keto acids can be used by many cells when glucose and fatty acids are not readily available (e.g., fasting). Insulin stimulates the uptake of glucose into cells, where it is stored in the form of glycogen (especially in the liver and skeletal muscle). It also stimulates fat synthesis and inhibits lipolysis, thus storing fatty acids as triglycerides (fatty acid metabolism to keto acids is also inhibited). Finally, insulin stimulates the uptake of amino acids into cells and their storage as protein. The net effect is that blood levels of glucose and keto acids decrease.

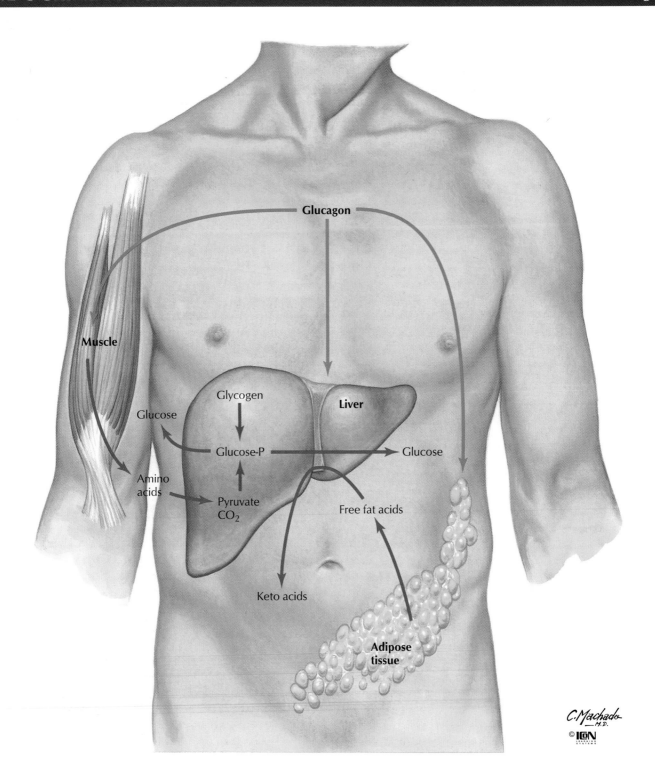

FIGURE 8.21 ACTIONS OF GLUCAGON

Glucagon is a fuel-mobilization hormone. It acts on the liver to break down glycogen and stimulates hepatic gluconeogenesis from amino acids. The effect of these actions is to increase the blood glucose concentration. Glucagon also acts on adipose tissue to stimulate lipolysis and the release of fatty acids. Metabolism of the fatty acids by the liver produces keto acids. Amino acids are released from muscle in response to glucagons and are converted to glucose in the liver by gluconeogenesis. The net effect of glucagon is that glucose, fatty acid, and keto acid levels in the blood increase.

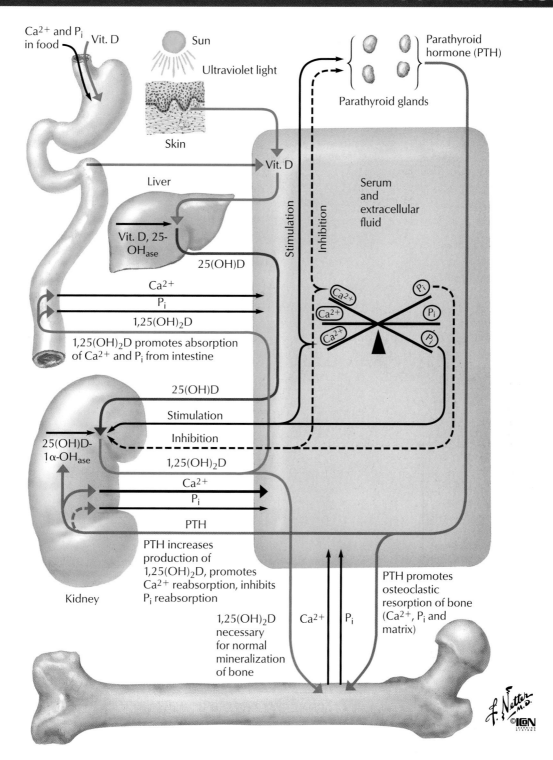

FIGURE 8.22 PARATHYROID HORMONE

The parathyroid glands secrete parathyroid hormone (PTH) in response to a decrease in the ionized [Ca^{2+}] of the blood. PTH acts on bone to cause resorption and release of Ca^{2+}. Renal reabsorption of Ca^{2+} is also stimulated by PTH (see Figure 6.16). PTH alters vitamin D metabolism. Vitamin D is a sterol produced in the skin and absorbed from the diet. It undergoes metabolic conversions in the liver and kidneys. PTH acts on the kidneys to stimulate the conversion of 25(OH)-vitamin D to the active form of the hormone, 1,25-(OH)₂-vitamin D (an increase blood P_i also stimulates

this conversion). The increased levels of 1,25-(OH)₂-vitamin D in turn stimulate the intestinal absorption of Ca^{2+}. The net effect of these actions is that PTH increases the ionized [Ca^{2+}] of the blood. PTH also causes the release of phosphate (P_i) from the bone and enhances its absorption from the GI tract. However, much of this P_i is excreted in the urine, because PTH also decreases renal P_i reabsorption (see Figure 6.16). Thus, the [P_i] of the blood is not significantly changed.

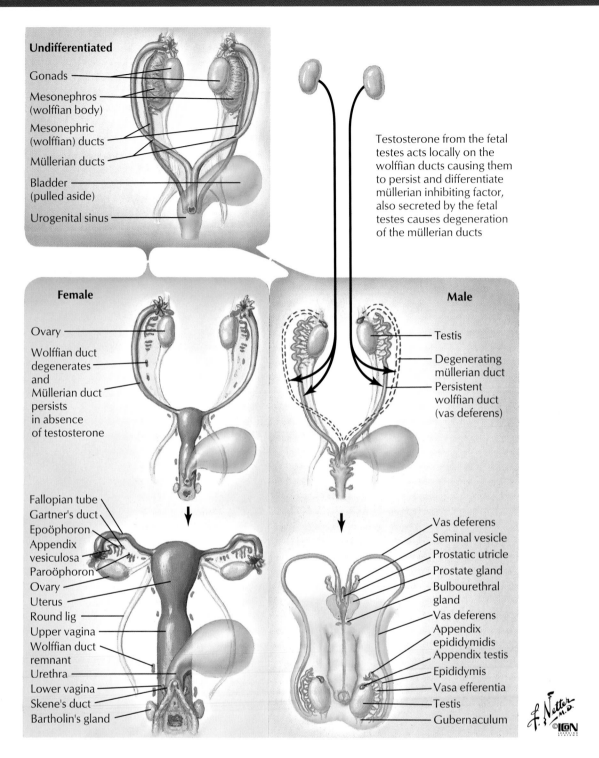

FIGURE 8.23   GONAD AND GENITAL DUCT FORMATION

Based on the expression of specific gene products under the control of the sex chromosomes (X and Y chromosomes), the undifferentiated gonads and duct system of the human embryo develop along the male or female lineage (the exact role of these gene products [SRY and DAX-1 genes] are still being investigated). In the presence of SRY gene expression (46XY complement of chromosomes), the fetal testes develop and produce testosterone, which acts locally on the mesonephric (wolffian) duct system (shown in red), which persists and develops into the efferent ductules, epididymis, vas defer-

ens, ejaculatory ducts, and the seminal vesicles. The paramesonephric (müllerian) ducts degenerate in response to a hormone called müllerian-inhibiting substance secreted by the fetal testes. In the absence of testosterone, the gonads of a normal female fetus (46XX complement of chromosomes) differentiate into paired ovaries, and the paramesonephric duct system (shown in blue in the left panels) persists while the mesonephric ducts degenerate. The paramesonephric ducts gives rise to paired uterine (fallopian) tubes, a midline uterus, and the upper portion of the vagina.

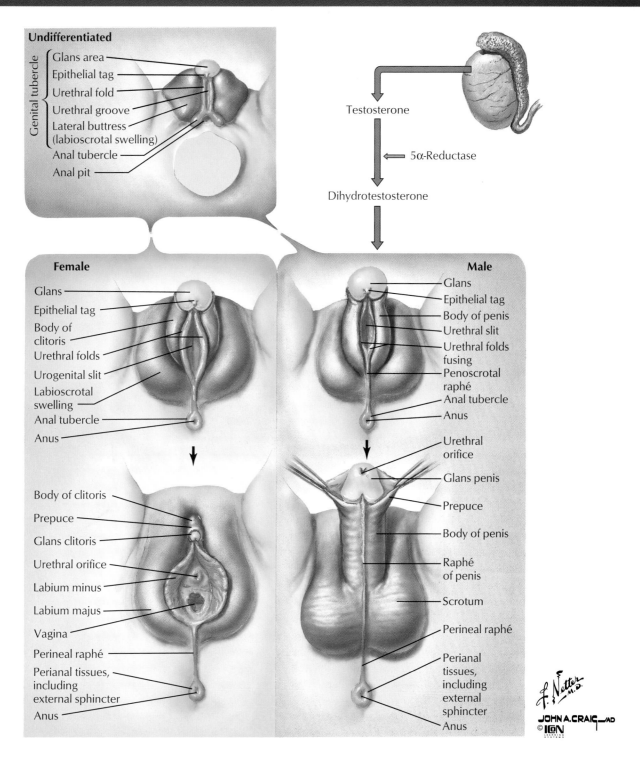

FIGURE 8.24   DIFFERENTIATION OF THE EXTERNAL GENITALIA

During early embryonic development, the external genitalia are undifferentiated and consist of tissue swellings comprised of the genital tubercle and urethral and anal folds. Under the influence of dihydrotestosterone, the genital tubercle elongates to form the phallus (glans) and normal male external genital development pro-ceeds. In the absence of testicular androgens, the undifferentiated genitalia develop into those of a normal female. The color scheme of this figure clearly shows the homologous structures of the external genitalia between the two sexes.

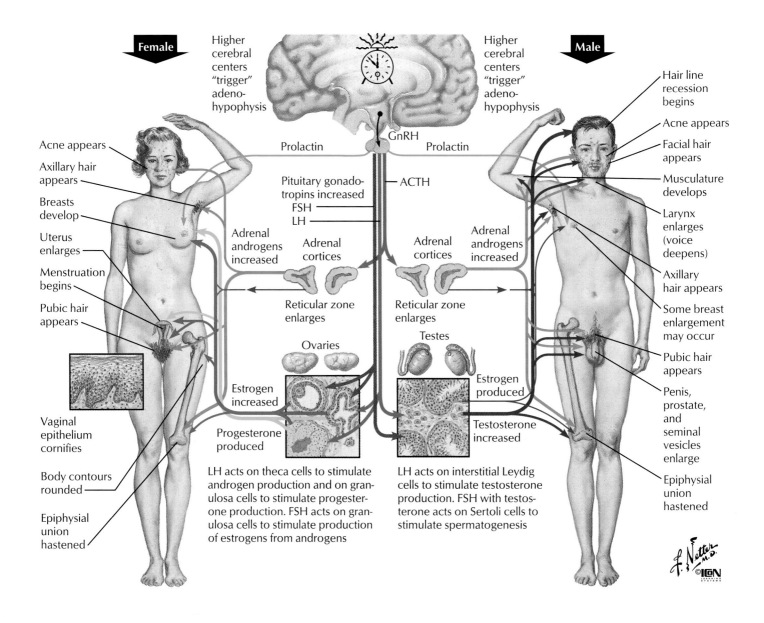

Female

Higher cerebral centers "trigger" adeno-hypophysis

Acne appears

Axillary hair appears

Breasts develop

Uterus enlarges

Menstruation begins

Pubic hair appears

Vaginal epithelium cornifies

Body contours rounded

Epiphysial union hastened

GnRH

Prolactin

Prolactin

Pituitary gonado-tropins increased
FSH
LH

ACTH

Adrenal androgens increased

Adrenal cortices

Reticular zone enlarges

Adrenal cortices

Adrenal androgens increased

Reticular zone enlarges

Ovaries

Testes

Estrogen increased

Estrogen produced

Progesterone produced

Testosterone increased

LH acts on theca cells to stimulate androgen production and on granulosa cells to stimulate progester-one production. FSH acts on granulosa cells to stimulate production of estrogens from androgens

LH acts on interstitial Leydig cells to stimulate testosterone production. FSH with testos-terone acts on Sertoli cells to stimulate spermatogenesis

Male

Higher cerebral centers "trigger" adeno-hypophysis

Hair line recession begins

Acne appears

Facial hair appears

Musculature develops

Larynx enlarges (voice deepens)

Axillary hair appears

Some breast enlargement may occur

Pubic hair appears

Penis, prostate, and seminal vesicles enlarge

Epiphysial union hastened

FIGURE 8.25   PUBERTY

One to two years before puberty, adrenal androgen levels increase (adrenarche). These adrenal androgens are responsible, in both sexes, for the early development of pubic and axillary hair and increased growth. At puberty, the hypothalamus increases the frequency and amount of gonadotropin-releasing hormone (GnRH) released. GnRH in turn stimulates the release of luteinizing hormone (LH) and follicle-stimulating hormone (FSH) by the anterior pituitary. In the male, LH acts on the interstitial Leydig cells of the testes to stimulate the production of testosterone. FSH together with testos-terone acts on the Sertoli cells of the testes, which are important for support and development of the spermatozoa. In the female, LH acts on both the theca and granulosa cells of the ovary. In response to LH, the theca cells produce androgens, which are then converted to estrogens by the granulosa cells. LH acts on the granulosa cells to stimulate progesterone production. FSH acts on the granulosa cells to stimulate the production of estrogens from androgens.

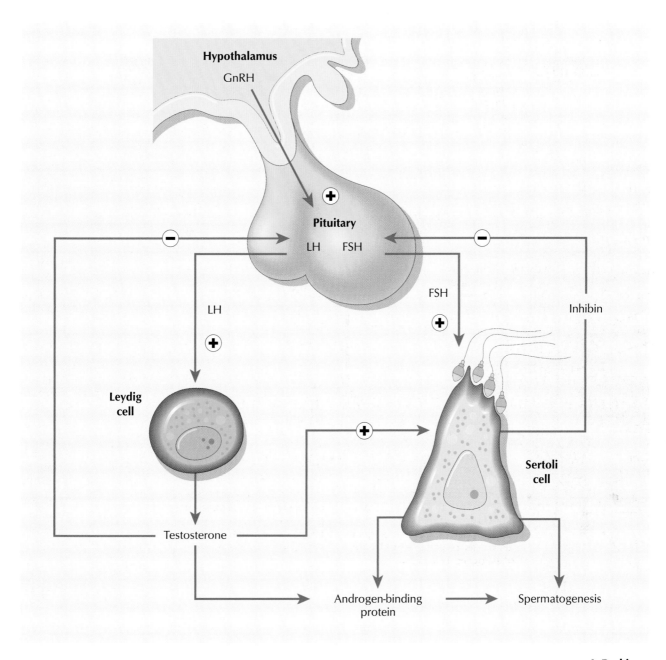

FIGURE 8.26   CONTROL OF TESTICULAR FUNCTION

The testes are under the control of luteinizing hormone (LH) and follicle-stimulating hormone (FSH), and their secretion from the anterior pituitary is controlled by gonadotropin-releasing hormone (GnRH) from the hypothalamus. LH acts on the interstitial Leydig cells to stimulate their production of testosterone. FSH acts on the Sertoli cells to stimulate their production of androgen-binding pro-tein, which then concentrates testosterone in the seminiferous tubules and thereby supports and promotes spermatogenesis. Testosterone provides negative feedback inhibition of LH release, whereas inhibin produced by the Sertoli cells provides negative feedback inhibition of FSH secretion.

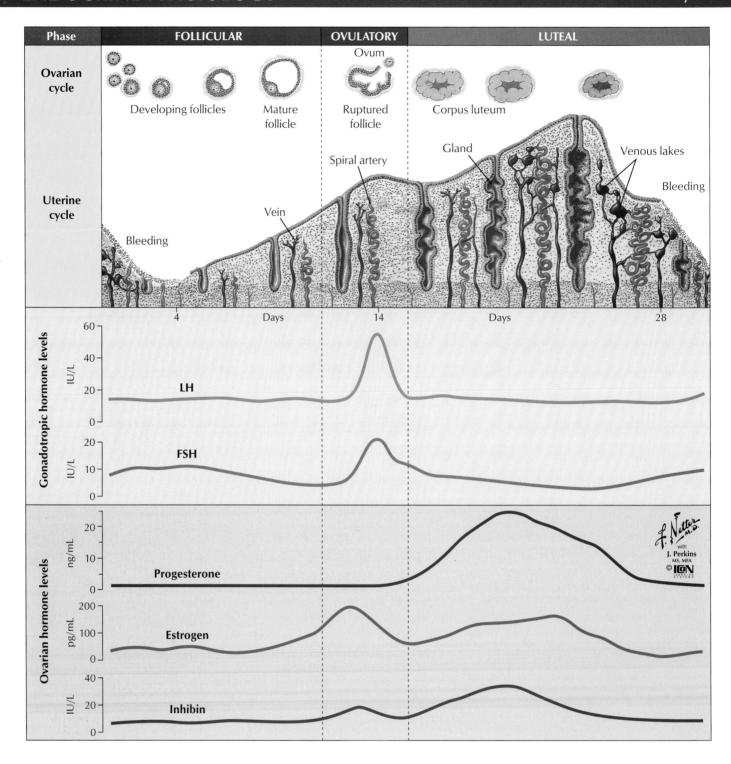

FIGURE 8.27 MENSTRUAL CYCLE

The menstrual cycle is divided into three phases: follicular, ovulatory, and luteal. The follicular phase begins during menses with the proliferation of the granulosa cells in a selected follicle. This is associated with rising levels of estradiol, and to a lesser extent, progestins, which feedback on both the hypothalamus and pituitary to stimulate (i.e., positive feedback) a surge in GnRH secretion followed by peaks in luteinizing (LH) and follicle-stimulating hormone (FSH) secretion, which then induce ovulation (see Figure 8.28).

Following ovulation, the follicular cells transform into the corpus luteum and produce large amounts of progesterone and estradiol. During this luteal phase, the granulosa cells also produce inhibin. Together, progesterone, estradiol, and inhibin feedback on the pituitary to suppress LH and FSH secretion (see Figure 8.28). In the absence of fertilization of the released egg, the corpus luteum regresses and menses begins.

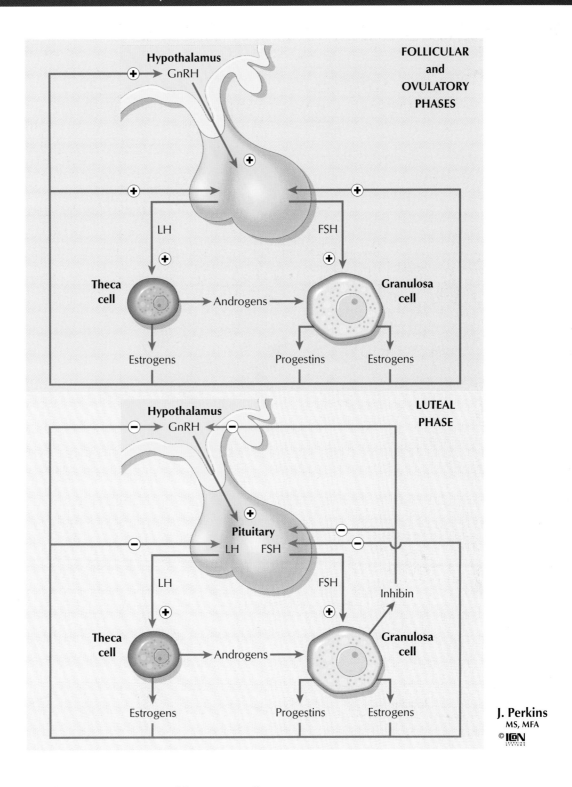

FIGURE 8.28   HORMONAL REGULATION OF THE MENSTRUAL CYCLE

Upper panel: During the follicular phase, the granulosa cells in a selected follicle proliferate and produce estradiol in response to follicle-stimulating hormone (FSH). At the same time, luteinizing hormone (LH) stimulates the theca cells to produce androgens. The androgens produced by the theca cells diffuse into the granulosa cells, where they are converted to estradiol. This leads to a large increase in estradiol production. The rising levels of estradiol, and to a lesser degree progestins (e.g., progesterone), feedback on both the hypothalamus and pituitary to stimulate (i.e., positive feedback) a surge in GnRH secretion followed by peaks in LH and FSH secretion, which then induce ovulation. *Lower panel:* Following ovulation, the remaining follicular cells transform into the corpus luteum in response to LH and produce large amounts of progesterone and estradiol. During this luteal phase, the granulosa cells also produce inhibin. Together, progesterone, estradiol, and inhibin feedback on the pituitary to suppress LH and FSH secretion. In the absence of fertilization of the released egg, the corpus luteum regresses and menses begins.

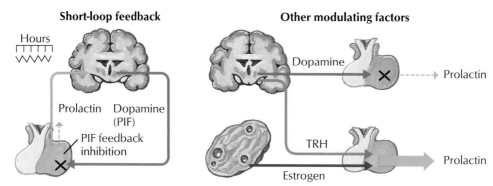

Short-loop feedback

Other modulating factors

Prolactin-inhibiting factor (PIF), thought to be dopamine, modulates prolactin secretion. Elevated prolactin levels increase PIF secretion and cause feedback inhibition of prolactin secretion (short-loop feedback inhibition). Estrogen and TRH stimulate prolactin secretion

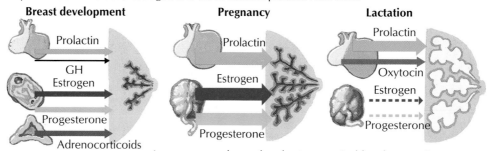

Breast development

Pregnancy

Lactation

Prolactin, along with GH, estrogen, progesterone, and adrenocorticoids, is necessary for breast development

In pregnancy, elevated prolactin, estrogen, and progesterone increase alveolobular development. High estrogen levels inhibit lactation

Sudden decrease in estrogen and progesterone in presence of prolactin results in milk production. Oxytocin stimulates milk release

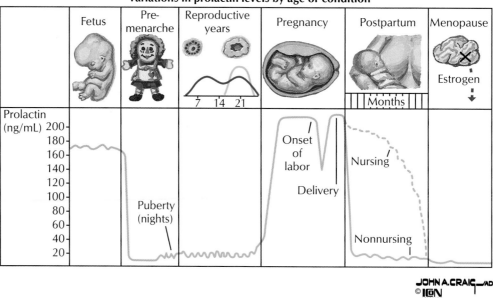

Variations in prolactin levels by age or condition

FIGURE 8.29 LACTATION

The role of prolactin in breast development, pregnancy, and lactation is summarized in this figure. Although prolactin is under dual hypothalamic control, it is unique because its secretion is under the inhibitory control of dopamine (PIF). *Abbreviation: GH, Growth hormone.*

INDEX

INDEX

In those instances where original artwork by Dr. Netter was not available to illustrate important physiological principles, the authors designed new figures and summary charts, which in some instances were based on figures and concepts presented in other sources. The authors gratefully acknowledge the following publications, which contain figures, charts, and diagrams that served as source materials for the design of these new figures and charts. "We are greatly indebted to our fellow scientists and educators."

Chart 1.1: Bourne HR et al. The GTPase superfamily: a conserved switch for diverse cell functions. *Nature.* 1990; 348:125; Chart 1.2 and Figures 4.9–4.11, 8.1, 8.2, and 8.28: Costanzo LS. *Physiology.* Philadelphia: W.B. Saunders; 1998; Figures 1.7 and 8.1: Cooper GM. *The Cell—A Molecular Approach.* 2nd ed. Washington, DC: ASM Press, Washington D.C., and Sinauer Associates, Inc., Sunderland, MA, 2000; Charts 2.1–2.3 and Figures 3.6, 3.9, 4.1, 4.9–4.14, 4.18, 4.19, 4.22, 5.12, 5.22, 5.26, 5.27, 6.8, 6.13–6.18, 7.6, 7.7, 7.11, 7.14, 7.25, 7.27, 7.34, 7.38, 8.1, 8.7, 8.9, 8.10, 8.13, 8.19–8.21, 8.26, and 8.28: Berne RM, Levy MN, eds. *Principles of Physiology.* 3rd ed. St. Louis: Mosby; 2000; Figure 2.3: Martini FH, Timmons MJ, McKinley MP. *Human Anatomy.* 3rd ed. Upper Saddle River, NJ: Prentice Hall; 2000; Figure 4.1: Despopoulos A, Silbernagl S. *Color Atlas of Physiology.* 4th ed. New York: Thieme Medical Publishers; 1991; Figure 4.5: Hille B. *Ionic Channels in Excitable Membranes.* 2nd ed. Sunderland, MA: Sinauer Associates; 1992; Figures 4.15, 4.20, 5.23, 6.8, and 6.13–6.18: Koeppen B, Stanton B. *Renal Physiology.* 3rd ed. St. Louis: Mosby; 2001; Figures 4.18 and 4.19: Heesch CM. Reflexes that control cardiovascular function. *Adv Physiol Educ.* 1999;22:S234; Figures 5.23, 5.26, and 5.27: Levitzky MG. *Pulmonary Physiology.* 5th ed. New York: McGraw-Hill; 1999; Figures 5.23, 5.26, and 5.27: West JB: *Pulmonary Physiology and Physiology—An Integrated Case-Based Approach.* Philadelphia: Lippincott Williams & Wilkins; 2001; Figures 7.8, 7.14, 7.25, and 7.34: Johnson LR. *Gastrointestinal Physiology.* 6th ed. St. Louis: Mosby; 2001; Figure 7.34: Montrose MH et al. Electrolyte secretion and absorption: small intestine and colon. In: Yamada T, ed. *Textbook of Gastroenterology.* 3rd ed. Philadelphia: Lippincott Williams & Wilkins; 1999; Figure 7.38: Andreas R, Hediger M. *Curr Opin Gastroenterol.* 2001;17:177; Figures 8.1, 8.7, 8.9, 8.10, 8.13, 8.19, 8.26, and 8.28: Porterfield SP. Endocrine Physiology. 2nd ed. St. Louis: Mosby; 2001; Figures 8.20 and 8.21: Marks DB et al. *Basic Medical Biochemistry—A Clinical Approach.* Philadelphia: Williams & Wilkins; 1996; Figure 8.27: Johnson LR. *Essential Medical Physiology.* 2nd ed. Philadelphia: Lippincott-Raven; 1998.